Principles
for
Nurse Staffing

WITH ANNOTATED BIBLIOGRAPY

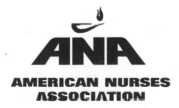

ANA

**AMERICAN NURSES
ASSOCIATION**

Library of Congress Cataloging-in-Publication Data

Principles for nurse staffing : annotated bibliography / compiled
by Rita Munley Gallager, Katherine A. Kany.
    p. cm.
    ISBN 1-55810-144-6 (pbk.)
    1. Nursing--Administration Bibliography. 2. Nursing
services--Personnel management Bibliography. 3. Nurses--Supply and
demand Bibliography. 4. Manpower planning Bibliography. I.
Gallagher, Rita Munley. II. Kany, Katherine A. III. American
Nurses Association.
    RT89.3 .P77 1999
362.1'73'0683--dc21   99-19077
                                                         CIP

Published by American Nurses Publishing
600 Maryland Avenue, SW
Suite 100 West
Washington, DC 20024-2571

ISBN 1-55810-144-6

9902AB   1.5M   03/99

Acknowledgments

EXPERT PANEL

Leah Curtin, ScD, RN, FAAN
Jacqueline Dienemann, PhD, RN, CNAA, FAAN
Christine Kovner, PhD, RN, FAAN
Mary Elizabeth Mancini, MSN, RN, CNA, FAAN
RADM Carolyn Beth Mazzella, MS, MPA, RN
RADM Kathryn Lothschuetz Montgomery, PhD, RN, CNAA
Judith Shindul-Rothschild, PhD, RN, CS
Julie Sochalski, PhD, RN, FAAN
Margaret D. Sovie, PhD, RN, FAAN
Joyce Verran, PhD, RN, FAAN

OTHER PARTICIPANTS

Cathy Coles, MSN, RN
Denise Geolot, PhD, RN, FAAN
Judy Goldfarb, MA, RN
Cheryl Jones, PhD, RN, CNAA
Lorraine Tulman, DNSc, RN, FAAN

Principles for Nurse Staffing adopted by ANA Board of Directors, November 24, 1998

Annotated bibliography compiled by Rita Munley Gallagher, PhD, RN, C, and Katherine A. Kany, BS, RN

Reviewed and revised January 11, 1999

Principles for Nurse Staffing

PATIENT CARE UNIT RELATED

- Appropriate staffing levels for a patient care unit reflect analysis of individual and aggregate patient needs.
- There is a critical need to either retire or seriously question the usefulness of the concept of nursing hours per patient day (HPPD).
- Unit functions necessary to support delivery of quality patient care must also be considered in determining staffing levels.

STAFF RELATED

- The specific needs of various patient populations should determine the appropriate clinical competencies required of the nurse practicing in that area.
- Registered nurses must have nursing management support and representation at both the operational level and the executive level.
- Clinical support from experienced RNs should be readily available to those RNs with less proficiency.

INSTITUTION/ORGANIZATION RELATED

- Organizational policy should reflect an organizational climate that values registered nurses and other employees as strategic assets and exhibit a true commitment to filling budgeted positions in a timely manner.
- All institutions should have documented competencies for nursing staff, including agency or supplemental and traveling RNs, for those activities that they have been authorized to perform.
- Organizational policies should recognize the myriad needs of both patients and nursing staff.

Contents

1. Introduction

Adequate nurse staffing is critical to the delivery of quality patient care. Identifying and maintaining the appropriate number and mix of nursing staff is a problem experienced by nurses at every level in all settings. Regardless of organizational mission, tempering the realities of cost containment and cyclical nursing shortages with the priority of safe, quality care has been difficult, in part, because of the paucity of empirical data to guide decision making. Since 1994, the recognition of this critical need for such empirical data has driven many American Nurses Association (ANA) activities, including identification of nursing-sensitive indicators, establishment of data collection projects using these indicators within the state nurses associations, and the provision of ongoing lobbying at federal and state levels for inclusion of these data elements within state and national data collection activities. In 1996, the Institute of Medicine produced its report *The Adequacy of Nurse Staffing in Hospitals and Nursing Homes* (Wunderlich, Sloan, and Davis 1996), in which it too recognized the need for such data. Despite these efforts, heightened and more immediate attention to issues related to the adequacy of nurse staffing is needed to ensure the provision of safe, quality nursing care.

2. Policy Statements

- Nurse staffing patterns and the level of care provided should not depend on the type of payor.
- Evaluation of any staffing system should include quality of work life outcomes as well as patient outcomes.
- Staffing should be based on achieving quality of patient care indices, meeting organizational outcomes, and ensuring that the quality of the nurse's work life is appropriate.

On April 1 and June 20, 1998, ANA convened a panel of experts in nursing practice and health services research to assist ANA in understanding and addressing issues related to staffing. The expertise of the panel was supplemented by representatives of organizations having significant interest in ANA's perspectives on nurse staffing. In their deliberations, the panel members described how changes in the delivery of health care have dramatically increased the complexity of the registered nurse's (RN's) role; have caused the exodus of more experienced (frequently more highly paid) nurses from acute care facilities and other settings; and have often resulted in a decrease in nursing management positions, historically strong advocates for patient[1] care priorities and for nursing staff. These concerns are made more significant in view of what many believe is the onset of yet another shortage of RNs.

During deliberations, the panel determined that consideration of nurse-to-patient ratios as a method for ascertaining staffing lacks any significant scientific support; therefore, panel members focused on the need to look at staffing with a different unit of analysis that would reflect the overall flow of activity of the patient care unit (a unit-based measurement) rather than the traditional nursing hour per patient day (HPPD). Adequate staffing is based on the complexity of care required by the patients, patient antecedents (including precipitating events, episode of care, intensity, and so forth), volume, and transactional issues. This combination of issues should serve as the foundation for staffing decisions and include the following considerations:

- The public perceives that quality of care in hospitals is tightly linked to adequate nursing staff. It believes the replacement of RN staff with lesser prepared licensed and unlicensed assistive personnel (UAP) is profit-motivated and indicative of a reversal of health care priorities (American Hospital Association 1997).
- Physicians support the increased use of RNs so that quality of care will be ensured (Gordon and Baer 1994).
- The cost, quality, and accessibility of care are improved when continuity of nursing care is ensured.
- Institutions differ by type, ownership, and mission (e.g., academic health centers, rural hospitals, public hospitals, for-profit agencies, and so forth). Those distinct differences must be taken into account when developing staffing patterns responsive to specific patient needs and organizational context.
- "Staffing," as both a budgeting process and the establishment of an overall structure to meet and anticipate care needs, must not be confused with the concept of "staffing," as the reality of managing available human resources on a shift-to-shift basis.
- Staffing levels must be sufficient to meet normal exigencies such as vacations, census variations, patient acuity changes, orientation of new or temporary staff, continuing education to maintain competencies of the staff overall, and nurse participation in agency governance.
- The practice environment must take into consideration the level of active involvement (both direct and indirect) and the professional complexity of the role of the RN to be conducive to the provision of quality care (Murphy 1993).

---

[1]". . . the recipients of nursing care are individuals, groups, families or communities . . . the individual recipient of nursing care can be referred to as patient, client, or person . . . The term 'patient' is used throughout to provide consistency and brevity. . . ." (ANA 1995).

- To create an environment conducive to providing quality care, nurses and the profession of nursing must be actively represented by an RN at all levels of the organization, including the executive level both within the institution itself and at the system level in multi-institution systems (Mintzberg 1996).
- To ensure the provision of quality care, the individual nurse must be responsible and accountable for independent decision making. As such, the RN must have the necessary authority as well as adequate time to plan, communicate, and engage in collegial relationships with all members of the health care team.

Beyond these considerations, principles for examining appropriate staffing levels at both the macro (budget and organizational) and micro (shift-to-shift) organizational levels have been developed. These principles, presented in the next section, can serve as the basis for the development of best practice models. The principles are targeted to three distinct areas and their evaluation: patient care unit (defined as a cluster—not necessarily geographically contiguous—of patients receiving care from the same general group of individuals); staff; and institution/organization.

3. Principles for Nurse Staffing

The nine principles identified by the expert panel for nurse staffing are listed below. A discussion of each of the three categories follows the list.

PATIENT CARE UNIT RELATED

- **Appropriate staffing levels for a patient care unit reflect analysis of individual and aggregate patient needs.**
- **There is a critical need to either retire or seriously question the usefulness of the concept of nursing hours per patient day (HPPD).**
- **Unit functions necessary to support delivery of quality patient care must also be considered in determining staffing levels.**

STAFF RELATED

- **The specific needs of various patient populations should determine the appropriate clinical competencies required of the nurse practicing in that area.**
- **Registered nurses must have nursing management support and representation at both the operational level and the executive level.**
- **Clinical support from experienced RNs should be readily available to those RNs with less proficiency.**

INSTITUTION/ORGANIZATION RELATED

- **Organizational policy should reflect an organizational climate that values registered nurses and other employees as strategic assets and exhibit a true commitment to filling budgeted positions in a timely manner.**
- **All institutions should have documented competencies for nursing staff, including agency or supplemental and traveling RNs, for those activities that they have been authorized to perform.**
- **Organizational policies should recognize the myriad needs of both patients and nursing staff.**

DISCUSSION OF PRINCIPLES

Patient Care Unit Related

There is a critical need to either retire or seriously question the usefulness of the concept of nursing HPPD. It is becoming increasingly clear that when determining nursing hours of care, one size (or formula) does *not* fit all. In fact, staffing is most appropriate and meaningful when it is predicated on a measure of unit intensity that takes into consideration the aggregate population of patients and the associated roles and responsibilities of nursing staff. Such a unit of measure must be operationalized to take into consideration the totality of the patients for whom care is being provided. It must not be predicated on a simple quantification of the needs of the "average" patients but must also include the "outliers." The following critical factors must be considered in the determination of appropriate staffing (see Table 1):

- Number of patients,
- Levels of intensity of the patients for whom care is being provided,

TABLE 1. MATRIX FOR STAFFING DECISION MAKING	
Items	**Elements and Definitions**
Patients	Patient characteristics and number of patients for whom care is being provided
Intensity of unit and care	Individual patient intensity; across-the-unit intensity (taking into account the heterogeneity of settings); variability of care; admisions, discharges, and transfers; and volume
Context	Architecture (geographic dispersion of patients, size and layout of individual patient rooms, arrangement of entire patient care unit(s), and so forth); technology (beepers, cellular phones, computers); same unit or cluster of patients
Expertise	Learning curve for individuals and groups of nurses; staff consistency, continuity, and cohesion; cross-training; control of practice; involvement in quality improvement activities; professional expectations; preparation and experience

- Contextual issues including architecture and geography of the environment and available technology, and
- Level of preparation and experience of those providing care.

Appropriate staffing levels for a patient care unit reflect analysis of individual and aggregate patient needs. The following specific patient physical and psychosocial considerations should be taken into account:

- Age and functional ability,
- Communication skills,
- Cultural and linguistic diversities,
- Severity and urgency of admitting condition,
- Scheduled procedure(s),
- Ability to meet health care requisites,
- Availability of social supports, and
- Other specific needs identified by the patient and by the registered nurse.

Unit functions necessary to support delivery of quality patient care must also be considered in determining staffing levels:

- Unit governance,
- Involvement in quality measurement activities,
- Development of critical pathways, and
- Evaluation of practice outcomes.

Staff Related

The specific needs of various patient populations should determine the clinical competencies required of the nurse. Role responsibilities and competencies of each nursing staff member should be well articulated, well defined, and documented at the operational level (Aiken, Smith, and Lake 1994). Registered nurses must have nursing management support and representation (first-line manager) at both the operational level and the executive level (nurse executive) (Aiken, Smith, and Lake 1994). Clinical support from experienced RNs should be readily available to RNs with less proficiency (McHugh et al. 1996). The following nurse characteristics should be taken into account when determining patient care unit staffing:

- Experience with the population being served;
- Level of experience (novice to expert);
- Education and preparation, including certification;
- Language capabilities;
- Tenure on the unit;

- Level of control of practice environment;
- Degree of involvement in quality initiatives;
- Measure of immersion in activities such as nursing research that add to the body of nursing knowledge;
- Measure of involvement in interdisciplinary and collaborative activities regarding patient needs in which the nurse takes part; and
- The number and competencies of clinical and nonclinical support staff the RN must collaborate with and supervise.

Institution/Organization Related

Organizational policy should reflect an organizational climate that values RNs and other employees as strategic assets and exhibits a true commitment to filling budgeted positions in a timely manner. In addition, personnel policies should reflect the agency's concern for employees' needs and interests (McClure et al. 1983).

All institutions should have documented competencies for nursing staff, including agency or supplemental and traveling RNs, for those activities that they have been authorized to perform (Joint Commission on the Accreditation of Healthcare Organizations 1998). When floating between units occurs, there should be a systematic plan in place for cross-training of staff to ensure competency (Joint Commission on the Accreditation of Healthcare Organizations 1998). Adequate preparation, resources, and information should be provided for those involved at all levels of decision making. Opportunities must be provided for individuals to be involved to the maximum amount possible in making the decisions that affect them (Williams and Howe 1994). Finally, any use of disincentives for reporting near misses and errors should be eliminated to foster continuous quality improvement (Leape 1994).

In addition, the organizational policies should recognize the myriad needs of both patients and nursing staff and provide the following:

- *Effective* and *efficient* support services (transport, clerical, housekeeping, laboratory, and so forth) to reduce time away from patient care and to reduce the need for the RN to engage in "re-work" (Prescott et al. 1991);
- Access to timely, accurate, relevant information provided by communication technology that links clinical, administrative, and outcome data;
- Sufficient orientation and preparation including nurse preceptors and nurse experts to ensure RN competency;
- Preparation specific to technology used in providing patient care;
- Necessary time to collaborate with and supervise other staff;
- Support in ethical decision making;
- Sufficient opportunity for care coordination and arranging for continuity of care and patient and family education;
- Adequate time for coordination and supervision of UAP by RNs;
- Processes to facilitate transitions during work redesign, mergers, and other major changes in work life (Bridges 1991);
- The right for staff to report unsafe conditions or inappropriate staffing without personal consequence; and
- A logical method for determining staffing levels and skill mix.

4. Evaluation

Adequate numbers of staff are necessary to reach a minimum level of quality patient care services. Ongoing evaluation and benchmarking related to staffing are necessary elements in the provision of quality care. At a minimum, this should include collection and analysis of nursing-sensitive indicators (ANA 1997) and their correlation with other patient care trends. It has been shown that the quality of work life has an effect on the quality of care delivered. Therefore, on an ongoing basis, the following trends should be evaluated:

- Work-related staff illness and injury rates (Shogren and Calkins 1995);
- Turnover/vacancy rates;
- Overtime rates;
- Rate of use of supplemental staffing;
- Flexibility of human resource policies and benefit packages;
- Evidence of compliance with applicable federal, state, and local regulations; and
- Levels of nurse staff satisfaction.

Staffing should be such that the quality of patient care is maintained, the quality of organizational outcomes are met, and the quality of nurses' work life is acceptable. **Changes in staffing levels, including changes in the overall number and/or mix of nursing staff, should be based on analysis of standardized, nursing-sensitive indicators.** The effect of these changes should be evaluated using the same criteria. Caution must be exercised in the interpretation of data related to staffing levels and patterns and patient outcomes in the absence of consistent and meaningful definitions of the variables for which data are being gathered.

5. Recommendations

Shifting the nursing paradigm away from an industrial model to a professional model would move the industry and organizations away from the technical approach of measuring time and motion to one that examines myriad aspects of using knowledge workers to provide quality care. This shift would spell the end to the "nurse-is-a-nurse-is-a-nurse" mentality by focusing on the complexity of unit activities and level(s) of nurse competency needed to provide quality patient care. To facilitate this shift, ANA makes the following recommendations:

- A distinct standardized definition of unit intensity must be developed. Factors to be taken into consideration in the development of such a definition include
  - Number of patients within the unit;
  - Levels of intensity of *all* of the patients for whom care is being provided;
  - Contextual issues including architecture and geography of the environment and available technology; and
  - Level of preparation and experience (i.e., competency) of those providing care.

- Data should be gathered to address the relationship between staffing and patient outcomes including but not limited to
  - Improvement in health status;
  - Achievement of appropriate self-care;
  - Demonstration of health-promoting behaviors;
  - Patient length of stay or visit;
  - Health-related quality of life;
  - Patient perception of being well cared for; and
  - Symptom management based on guidelines (Mitchell et al. 1997).

6. References

Aiken, L. H., Smith, H. L., and Lake, E. T. (1994). Lower Medicare mortality among a set of hospitals known for good nursing care. *Medical Care* 32(8):771–87.

American Hospital Association. (1997). *Reality Check: Public Perception of Health Care and Hospitals.* Chicago: American Hospital Association.

American Nurses Association. (1995). *Nursing's Social Policy Statement.* Washington, DC: American Nurses Association.

American Nurses Association. (1997). *Implementing Nursing's Report Card: A Study of RN Staffing, Length of Stay and Patient Outcomes.* Washington, DC: American Nurses Association.

Bridges, W. (1991). *Managing Transitions: Making the Most of Change.* Reading, MA: Addison-Wesley Publishing.

Gordon, S., and Baer, E. D. (1994, December 6). Fewer nurses to answer the buzzer. *The New York Times,* p. A23.

Joint Commission on the Accreditation of Healthcare Organizations. (1998, January). *Comprehensive Accreditation Manual for Hospitals: The Official Handbook.* Oakbrook Terrace, IL: The Joint Commission on the Accreditation of Healthcare Organizations.

Leape, L. (1994). Error in medicine. *Journal of the American Medical Association* 272(23):1851–57.

McClure, M. L., Poulin, M. A., Sovie, M. D., and Wandelt, M. A. (1983). *Magnet Hospitals: Attraction and Retention of Professional Nurses.* Kansas City, MO: American Nurses Association.

McHugh, M., West, P., Assatly, C., Duprat, L., Howard, L., Niloff, J., Waldo, K., Wandel, J., and Clifford, J. (April 1996). Establishing an interdisciplinary patient care team. *Journal of Nursing Administration* 26(4):21–27.

Mintzberg, H. (1996, July–August). Musings on management. *Harvard Business Review,* 61–67.

Mitchell, P. H., Heinrich, J., Moritz, P., and Hinshaw, A. S. (1997). Outcome measures and care delivery systems: Introduction and purposes of conference. *Medical Care: Official Journal of the Medical Care Section, American Public Health Association* 35(11 Supplement):NS1–NS5.

Murphy, E. C. (1993). *Cost-Driven Downsizing in Hospitals: Implications for Mortality.* Amherst, NY: E.C. Murphy.

Prescott, P., Ryan, J. W., Soeken, K. L., Castorr, A. H., Thompson, K. O., and Phillips, C. Y. (1991). The patient intensity for nursing index: A validity assessment. *Research in Nursing Health* 14:213–21.

Shogren, B., and Calkins, A. (1995). *Minnesota Nurses Association Research Project on Occupational Injury/Illness in Minnesota Between 1990–1994.* St. Paul, MN: The Minnesota Nurses Association.

Williams, T., and Howe, R. (1994). W. Edwards Deming and total quality management: An interpretation for nursing practice. *Journal for Healthcare Quality* 14(2):36–39.

Wunderlich, G. S., Sloan, F. A., and Davis, C. K. (1996). *Nursing Staff in Hospitals and Nursing Homes: Is it Adequate?* Washington, DC: National Academy Press.

7. Annotated Bibliography

The following annotated bibliography provides background information on which the principles are based.

_____. (1998). **Slants & trends.** *Legislative Network for Nurses* 15(24):185.

This article reports on recommended guidelines for minimum staffing levels in long-term care facilities. The guidelines were promulgated by attendees at the National Citizen's Coalition for Nursing Home Reform's conference. The group's perspective is that these guidelines should be drafted in state statutes.

The article contains no bibliography, graphs, or charts.

_____. (1998). **National Council studies employment rate, work setting of newly licensed nurses.** *Issues* 19(1):7–9.

The National Council (of State Boards of Nursing) engages in job analysis of newly licensed RNs and licensed practical/vocational (LPN/VNs) on a three-year cycle. The latest RN study was completed in July 1996; the LPN/VN study was performed in July 1997.

This article details the methodology for performing the study and provides statistical information about the rate of employment and the work settings of newly licensed nurses who were surveyed between July 1996 and October 1997.

The results highlight differences in the rates and reasons for unemployment among newly licensed LPN/VNs and RNs. Although the primary reason for unemployment within the RN group is an inability to find a position, this does not apply to the LPN/VN respondents. Unlike the RNs surveyed, a seasonal variation in employment rates appears to exist within the LPN/VN respondents.

The primary employment site for LPN/VNs remains the long-term care setting, while that for RNs is in acute care settings. Throughout the eighteen months of this study, the differences noted, although not statistically significant, demonstrate the variability in the availability of jobs for these two licensure groups in various sections of the market. In addition, an interaction appears to exist between the availability of employment in a specific work setting and the type of licensee employed.

A six-item bibliography is included. There are two tables: Reasons newly licensed LPN/VNs were not employed in nursing and reasons newly licensed RNs were not employed in nursing. Two figures detail the employment settings of newly licensed LPN/VNs and newly licensed RNs.

_____. (1997). **Preparing patient care executives to manage complexity: An interview with Joyce A. Verran, PhD, RN, FAAN.** *Aspen's Advisor for Nurse Executives* 12(6):1, 3, 6.

The interview presents Dr. Verran's perspectives on the challenges inherent in the changes taking place in health care as they relate to the preparation of professional nurses. Verran points out that doctoral preparation will be required for nurse executives. She notes the primary importance of the qualifications and research involvement of the faculty to the preparation of graduate students in nursing administration.

The article contains no bibliography, graphs, or charts.

Aiken, L. (1995). Transformation of the nursing workforce. *Nursing Outlook* 43(5):201–209.

The article points out that nurses are not being used to their full potential in the current health care system. This shortcoming results in limited access to health care for some portions of the American public and in less than optimal care being provided at higher costs because RNs are prevented from fully participating. Both the public and professional nursing would benefit from reduction in these barriers.

The article includes a thirty-six-item bibliography. There are seven figures: Nurse-to-population ratio (per 100,000 population), 1950–1992; Percent change in nurse employment in selected areas, 1988–1992; Cumulative real case-mix change in hospitals, 1981–1992; Education of new nurses; Graduations from master's programs, actual and hypothetical, 1973–1991; Trends in Title VIII appropriations (in thousands); and Enrollment in master's programs by full-time status, United States, 1973–1992.

Aiken, L. H. (1990). Changing the future of hospital nursing. *IMAGE: The Journal of Nursing Scholarship* **22(2):72–78.**

This article makes the case that nursing cannot afford to turn a deaf ear to the persistent problems that undermine innovation and creativity in hospital nursing practice. As important as the broad agenda of nursing is to expanding community-based nursing practice, it is essential to most nurses and to the public they serve to persevere in their attempts to reform hospital nursing practice. This proposal calls for the development of additional career tracks in hospital nursing, most of which are predominantly clinical. The clinical career trajectories should be designed to approximate more closely the organization of medical care in hospitals and have the explicit goal of closer collaboration between medicine and nursing. The author notes that it will not be possible to reduce the number of nurses needed to provide hospital care unless substantial changes are made in the organization and delivery of nonnursing services in hospitals. In addition, the number of nurses could be reduced without adversely affecting the care of patients if additional administrative, secretarial, and clerical personnel were available. Greater creativity, the author states, could be used in developing safe and effective roles for assistants to whom nurses could delegate functions that need to be done in hospitals but do not require the time of a professional.

The article includes one table of nurse-to-population ratios in selected countries in 1984. The article also includes three figures depicting the supply of nurses from 1960 to 1988, hospital nurses' monthly wages in 1982 dollars from 1972 to 1989, and career tracks in hospital nursing. There is a forty-one-item bibliography. The author notes that overidentification with the concerns of management and preoccupation with the day-to-day operations of the institution divert nurses' time, attention, and perhaps even loyalties away from patients and away from the clinical challenges and common interests they share with physicians.

Aiken, L. H., and Salmon, M. E. (1994). Health care workforce priorities: What nursing should do now. *Inquiry* **31:318–329.**

This article appraises the adequacy of the aggregate supply of nurses and the appropriateness of their educational mix in view of anticipated changes in health care. The authors view the supply as adequate but the educational mix as deficient with regard to nurses with baccalaureate and higher degrees who will be in greatest demand in new and expanding roles. Five priority areas are identified in which nursing can make important contributions to improving health and health care: restructuring hospitals, improving primary care availability, contributing to the viability of academic health centers, improving care of the underserved, and redesigning the role of public health in a reformed health care system.

Two figures detailing full-time equivalent RNs employed in hospitals (1980 to 1992) and primary care practitioners: nurses and physicians (1992) are included. A table of estimated cost to Medicare of extending direct reimbursement to nurse practitioners (NPs) and physician assistants (PAs) as proposed in the *Health Security Act* is also included. There is a forty-five-item bibliography. This article calls for nursing to take a leadership role in the "reinventing" of public health to ensure that population-based community outreach by public health nurses remains a component of public health, at least until it can be demonstrated that the evolving infrastructure of health care reform has the capacity to do this in some other way.

Aiken, L. H., Smith, H. L., and Lake, E. T. (1994). Lower Medicare mortality among a set of hospitals known for good nursing care. *Medical Care* **32(8):771–787.**

This article reports on a study that investigated whether hospitals known to be good places to practice nursing have lower Medicare mortality than hospitals that are otherwise similar with respect to a variety of nonnursing organizational characteristics. The authors match a set of studies of thirty-nine "magnet" hospitals that, for reasons other than patient outcomes, have been singled out as hospitals known for good nursing care, with 195 hospitals controlling for hospital characteristics. The study found that the magnet hospitals, which embody a set of organizational attributes that nurses find desirable (and that are conducive to better patient care), have lower mortality than matched hospitals, which are similar along other organizational dimensions but are not known as settings that place a high institutional priority on nursing. Those familiar with the inner workings of hospitals will not be surprised that a relationship exists between the practice of nursing and the mortality experience of hospital patients. The connection between nursing and mortality rates dates as far back as the reforms in British hospitals made under Florence Nightingale during the Crimean War.

The "magnet" hospitals did differ from their matched controls in their nursing "skill mix," but this is not the explanation for the mortality differential. Based on adjunct studies of the magnet hospitals, the authors are inclined to attribute this difference to hospital-level differences in the organization of nursing care. The broader conclusion is that such organizational factors are important in understanding why some hospitals achieve better patient outcomes than others.

The article contains three tables. One table presents a comparison from two studies of the presence of autonomy, control, and relations with physicians as assessed by nurses for magnet and other hospitals. The second table outlines the characteristics of the study hospitals. The third presents estimated parameters for three models of hospital mortality. There is a fifty-nine-item bibliography. The article offers the potential for the organization of nursing services to provide a means for reducing hospital mortality.

Aiken, L. H., and Sochalski, J. (Eds.). (1997). Hospital restructuring in North America and Europe: Patient outcomes and workforce implications. *Medical Care: Official Journal of the Medical Care Section, American Public Health Association* **35 (10 Supplement).**

This supplement advances the debate related to the maintenance of excellent and affordable hospitals. The articles listed below discuss issues related to the quality or cost trade-offs inherent in health care today. The articles discuss the topics brought forward in the Bellagio conference on hospital restructuring, which sought to understand the restructuring of hospitals across a variety of countries. The supplement contains the following:

Aiken, L. H., and Fagin, C. M.	Preface
Clancy, C. M., and Gross, M. L.	Foreword
White, K. L.	Introduction: Hospital restructuring in North America and Europe

Hospital Systems Change

Sochalski, J., Aiken, L. H., and Fagin, C. M.	Hospital restructuring in the United States, Canada, and Western Europe: An outcomes research agenda
Maarse, H., Mur-Veeman, I., and Speeuwenberg, C.	The reform of hospital care in the Netherlands
Busse, R., and Schwartz, F.W.	Financing reforms in the German hospital sector: From full cost cover principle to prospective case fees
Harrison, A. J.	Hospitals in England: Impact of the 1990 National Health Service Reforms
Shamian, J., and Lightstone, E. Y.	Hospital restructuring initiatives in Canada
Decter, M. B.	Canadian hospitals in transformation

Hospital Outcomes Research

Silber, J. H., and Rosenbaum, P. R.	A spurious correlation between hospital mortality and complication rates: The importance of severity adjustment
Anderson, G. M.	Hospital restructuring and the epidemiology of hospital utilization: Recent experience in Ontario
McKee, M., and James, P.	Using routine data to evaluate quality of care in British hospitals
Bitzer, E. M., Dorning, H., Busse, R., and Schwartz, F. W.	Hospital outcomes research in Germany: Results from a retrospective survey among sickness fund beneficiaries

Hospital Restructuring: Impact on the Health Care Workforce

Baumgart, A. J.	Hospital reform and nursing labor market trends in Canada
Muller-Mundt, G.	Trends in hospital restructuring and impact on the workforce in Germany
Buchan, J., Hancock, C., and Rafferty, A. M.	Health sector reform and trends in the United Kingdom hospital workforce

Aiken, L. H., Sochalski, J., and Anderson, G. F. (1996, Winter). Downsizing the hospital nursing workforce. *Health Affairs* 15(4):88–92.

The authors reconcile nurses' perceptions that hospitals are reducing nurse staffing to unsafe levels with the dominant hospital management view that major restructuring of the hospital workforce, including nursing, is warranted. The article brings together empirical data from a number of sources to examine the overall trends in hospital employment and to determine the implications for current hospital restructuring activities as well as nurses' future job prospects. The authors take the position that perceptions of RN job reductions derive from several factors: the decline in the overall number of nursing personnel; the highly publicized actions at various institutions; and the rate of growth in the supply of RNs is outstripping job growth for RNs (particularly in certain geographic areas). The market for RNs has been reasonably self-correcting over time. Although the demand for RNs still appears to be strong, it is unclear whether graduating cohorts of 95,000 (the size of the class of 1994) will continue to be absorbed as hospital job growth is curtailed. The supply of RNs likely will be tempered in the future if job availability is reduced. If nurses' wages stagnate and fall relative to those of aides and LPNs, the demand for nurses in hospitals could increase to the point of exhausting what may appear to be an oversupply, resulting in the kinds of shortages of RNs experienced in the 1980s. Finally, the average age of the nursing workforce is increasing, suggesting that retirement could increase greatly over the long term, thus providing more job opportunities for new graduates. The biggest potential threat to nursing in the near term is not job availability. It is the possibility that in the quest to reduce spending, hospital management will implement poorly conceived re-engineering plans that could undermine nursing's best efforts to maintain the quality and safety of clinical care.

Two tables are within the article. Exhibit 1 presents the percentage of change in full-time-equivalent hospital personnel per 1,000 case mix-adjusted patient days between 1981 and 1993. Also detailed is the growth in full-time-equivalent hospital registered nurses per 100 case mix-adjusted average daily census. A twelve-item bibliography is contained within the endnotes. The article supports a prediction of an impending shortage of RNs.

American Hospital Association. (1997). *Reality Check: Public Perception of Health Care and Hospitals.* **Chicago: American Hospital Association.**

This report summarizes qualitative research done through focus groups convened across the United States to provide information regarding public perception toward health care in general and particularly about hospitals and the role they play in the changing world of health care delivery. Findings show that the public is deeply concerned and troubled about changes occurring in health care and hospitals. People feel a reduced accessibility to health care, as well as higher costs and lower quality. Those participating cited concerns with the competence of caregivers and the lack of personalized care. Of note in this report is the finding that the "key indicator" of quality of care was the adequacy of RNs.

American Nurses Association. (1997). *Implementing Nursing's Report Card: A Study of RN Staffing, Length of Stay and Patient Outcomes.* **Washington, DC: American Nurses Association.**

This study is a pilot project to ascertain the usefulness of observing a number of nursing's quality indicators. It uses three states (California, New York, and Massachusetts) for two years (1992, a year after the most recent nursing "shortage" in which requirements for nursing were high, and 1994, the latest year data was fully available) to meet the study's two main goals: to assess the feasibility of capturing the information necessary to develop specific nurse staffing and outcome measures for hospitals in those states with acceptable degrees of reliability and validity; and to statistically test the relationships between specific patient outcome indicators and nurse staffing.

The study's methodology was intended to quantify nurse staffing at the sample hospitals; quantify patient incidents and lengths of stay at the same hospitals; and measure the relationship among these sets of variables. Shorter lengths of stay were found to be highly correlated with higher nurse staffing per acuity-adjusted day. Patient morbidity indicators for preventable conditions—pressure ulcers, pneumonia, postoperative infections, and urinary tract infections—were found to be statistically significantly inversely related to RN skill mix, and to a smaller degree, nurse staffing per acuity-adjusted day; and nursing intensity weights by diagnosis-related groups (DRG) were statistically significantly positively correlated to differences in nurse staffing ratios per patient day in all three states.

The article contains twelve tables. The tables provide details on data sources, nursing percentage of worked hours by direct patient care cost center, nursing hours per day in hospitals with high versus low nursing intensity weights per day as well as diagnoses used to identify adverse outcomes. Other tables detail nurse staffing by hospital "teachingness" and setting. The article also includes tables that focus on nurse staffing by hospital metropolitan statistical area, the significance level correlations of dependent variables with one or more independent variables, geometric length of stay index, pressure ulcer adverse outcome rates, pneumonia, and postoperative infection and urinary tract infection adverse outcome rates. Three bibliographic entries are included within footnotes.

Barter, M., McLaughlin, F. E., and Thomas, S. (March April 1994). Use of unlicensed assistive personnel by hospitals. *Nursing Economic$* **12(2):82–87.**

This article reports on a survey of acute care hospitals to investigate the restructuring of nursing care services in acute care hospitals by the addition of unlicensed assistive personnel (UAP). Most unlicensed personnel in the hospitals studied were used in simple bedside care (84 percent), documented care only on graphic or flow sheets (75 percent), and were not consistently supervised by the same RN (97 percent). Of the 234 California hospitals surveyed, only 26 required a high school diploma and 29 percent of the hospitals preferred certification as a certified nursing assistant. Most (88 percent) of the hospitals provided less than 40 hours of classroom training for UAP. Less than 120 hours of on-the-job training was provided by most hospitals (99 percent), and data collected showed UAP were replacing LVNs in acute care hospitals. Findings suggest that the efficacy of this restructuring model was not established in advance of implementation and that standardized training and utilization policies also did not exist. The summary suggests that well-designed studies that measure patient outcomes, cost-effectiveness, and work satisfaction are needed to understand better the effect of UAP use in nursing care delivery systems.

This article contains five tables outlining sample hospitals, nursing care delivery models, amount of classroom instruction time provided to new UAP, amount of on-the-job training provided for new UAP, and cost of orientation for UAP. One figure shows trends in patient census and full-time equivalents. A fifteen-article bibliography is included. The article reinforces the importance of thoughtful evaluation and analysis of potential implications of restructuring nursing care delivery.

Bellandi, D. (1998, March 16). Healthcare industry gets clean bill of health. *Modern Healthcare,* **68–74.**

After a decade of dire predictions about the fate of the health care industry made by consultants, studies, and surveys, the outlook is bullish. The article contains no bibliography but has three charts: aggregate profits, drawn from American Hospital Association statistics; total spending and percent increase reported by the Health Care Financing Administration (HCFA); and estimation of what might have been reported by the Prospective Payment Assessment Commission (ProPAc).

Berland, A. (1990, May). Controlling workload. *Canadian Nurse,* **36–38.**

This article presents details of a policy, "Restriction of Admission to Nursing Units," that successfully addressed both budgetary and workload concerns. This policy recognized the experience of head nurses and the need to protect staff nurses from burnout. Under full restriction, no patients would be admitted no matter how many beds were unoccupied. Under partial restriction, no patients would be admitted until the number of unoccupied beds exceeded a defined number of restricted beds. A critical component in implementation of the policy was the emphasis on communication with medical staff. Initially, the policy required head nurses to document the patient care conditions that necessitated bed restrictions. Sent to the nursing director and the medical director of the unit, these documents were revealing. They not only described patient acuity but also explained to physicians some of the advanced nursing skills practiced by nurses at the bedside. Several dramatic effects emerged as a result of the new policy. First, the nursing division's use of overtime dropped dramatically to one-third the previous year's usage. Because overtime workers are paid time and a half, the savings were substantial. The division now spends considerably less on overtime than on staff development. Second, the hospital has continued to attract nurses. Third, and perhaps most important, staff nurses feel more in control of their workload.

The article has no figures, charts, or tables, although there is a three-item bibliography. The article points up the necessity of nursing administration supporting direct care providers.

Blegen, M. A., Goode, C. J., and Reed, L. (1998). Nurse staffing and patient outcomes. *Nursing Research* **47(1):43–50.**

Nursing research has shown that changes in nursing care delivery affect staff and organizational outcomes, but the attendant effect on client outcomes has not been thoroughly studied. This article discusses, at the nursing care unit level, the correlation among total hours of nursing care, RN skill mix, and adverse patient outcomes. The adverse outcomes included unit rates of medication errors, patient falls, skin breakdown, patient and family complaints, infections, and deaths. The relationships among staffing variables and outcome variables were identified, and multivariate analyses, controlling for patient acuity, were undertaken.

Units with higher average patient acuity had lower rates of medication errors and patient falls but higher rates of the other adverse outcomes. When the average patient acuity on the unit was controlled, the percentage of hours of care delivery by RNs was inversely related to the unit rates of medication errors, decubiti, and patient complaints. Total hours of care from all nursing personnel were directly related to the rates of decubiti, complaints, and mortality. A serendipitous finding was that the relationship between RN proportion of care was curvilinear; as the RN proportion increased, rates of adverse outcomes decreased up to 87.5 percent. Over that level, as RN proportion increased, the adverse outcome rates also increased. The higher the RN skill mix, the lower the incidence of adverse occurrences on inpatient care units.

The article has a thirty-seven-item bibliography. The article includes three tables: means, standard deviation (SD), and range of study variables; correlations for all study variables; and multiple regression models for all outcome variables.

Bodinsky, G. N. (1994). Developing a staffing model. *Gastroenterology Nursing* **17(2):72–75.**

This article outlines the importance of considering several factors before determining staffing. These factors include what constitutes an adequate level of care; appropriate staff mix; permanent versus temporary staff; and capacities in which all staff should be assigned. Use of a daily diary time study is useful in determining patient acuity, and listing direct and indirect care activities can be substituted for more expensive time study sampling and can be done by staff. Other important tools for determining staffing include using patient classification systems and using weighted scales for procedures. Findings support the value of all three approaches to determine and defend appropriate staff numbers and mix while continuing to evaluate each for their strengths and weaknesses.

This article contains eight tables listing information used in the development of a staffing model for an endoscopy unit. There is an eleven-item bibliography. The article provides thoughtful consideration of aspects important to the development of appropriate, unit-specific staffing.

Brewer, C. S. (1997). Through the looking glass: the labor market for registered nurses in the 21st century. *Nursing and Health Care Perspectives* **18(5):260–69.**

From the 1950s through the beginning of the 1990s, nurses had virtual employment security. Currently, the supply exceeds demand, and nursing student enrollments have declined. This article discusses the possible causes and identifies the rules of the market that can be used to predict the future of nursing. Reductions in reimbursement for health care services provided along with the rapid increase in managed care and competition with the industry have resulted in cost-cutting measures, many which have directly affected the nursing workforce. To meet the future head on, professional nurses will be required to have an understanding of the implications of economics on the profession.

A fifty-three-item bibliography is included. The article contains two tables (wage increases from 1991 to 1996 and total U.S. enrollments 1985 to 1995) and two figures (baccalaureate and graduation data 1992 to 1997 and total baccalaureate enrollment 1991 to 1996).

Carr-Hill, R. A., and Jenkins-Clarke, S. (1995). Measurement systems in principle and in practice: The example of nursing workload. *Journal of Advanced Nursing* **22:221–25.**

A rapid development of measurement systems has occurred in health services in the United Kingdom (UK) during recent years. This development has not always been accompanied by a thorough understanding of the phenomenon being measured and has rarely been based on any assessment of reliability or validity. A flagrant example of this process is the development of nursing workload measurement systems (NWMS). The estimates from four NWMS were examined in the study in this article. They were substantially different from each other, and the difference between any of the estimates and the actual nursing hours worked could not be explained in terms of any other aspect of the nursing process. No evidence exists that the NWMS deployed in the United Kingdom are anything more than a costly subterfuge without this kind of investigation of how they actually work in practice. It would be prudent to be wary about any of the measurement systems that have been proposed.

The article includes three tables. One presents total hours estimated according to different NWMS. The second table details the average proportion of outcomes achieved. The third presents estimates of over- and understaffing. A seventeen-item bibliography is included. The article notes that measurement systems, just like clinical procedure, must be tested for practicability, reliability, and validity before being adopted on a wide scale.

Carroll, P. (1998). Buyer beware? *Subacute Care Today* **1(5):24–28.**

As subacute care providers enter the era of prospective payment, managers and administrators will be looking to the hospital industry for examples of how to reduce costs. The acute care component of health care has been operating under a like system for more than ten years. Personnel costs seem to be the most likely to be cut because salaries and benefits are generally the largest budget items in any facility. However, replacing higher-cost, better-educated, and better-trained workers with lower-cost, lesser-educated, and lesser-trained workers has had mixed results in most hospitals.

The use of unlicensed assistive personnel (UAP) to reduce personnel costs has become the practice in hospitals during the past ten years as hospital administrators struggled with the difficulty of reducing the costs of delivering care to meet the reduction in reimbursements. UAP are hired and trained by the hospital, which also defines their scope of practice. There are no standards or standardized training programs for these workers.

The article proposes a more explicit term to describe these workers: noncredentialed assistive personnel (NCAP). The clarification is significant. A variety of highly skilled and prepared workers, including surgical technologists and, in some states, respiratory care practitioners (RCPs), have national credentials but are not licensed by the states. Technically, these individuals could be categorized as "unlicensed assistive personnel." However, the term UAP generally refers to workers who are not highly skilled or otherwise credentialed. The license is not the relevant factor; the clinical experience and preparation are. However, practitioners must be educated as to how to delegate appropriately. More important, facilities must use NCAPs to assist—not replace—clinicians.

The article contains one figure, which provides the National Council of State Boards of Nursing's perspective on delegation. The article also contains two references and a seven-item bibliography.

Cunningham, R. (1998, April 27). New Pew report stirs dialogue on future nursing workforce needs. *Medical & Health Perspectives,* **1–4.**

Much of the medical profession was outraged in 1995 when the Pew Health Professions Commission recommended closing 20 percent of the nation's medical schools and decreasing the number of physicians, nurses, and pharmacists by ten to twenty-five percent by the year 2005. The reduction in hospital excess capacity is moving unevenly from one region of the country to another, as is the attendant growth of care provision in ambulatory settings. The net result for professional nursing is uncertain. However, for workforce forecasters, the future holds nothing but ever-increasing risks.

This article does not include a bibliography. However, it contains one table, hospital and nursing home employees 1988–1994, from the Institute of Medicine/Bureau of Labor Statistics.

Davis, B. (1994). Effective utilization of a scarce resource: RNs. *Nursing Management* **25(2):78–80.**

Nursing costs are said to make up nearly half of a hospital's total budget, a situation exacerbated by the RN shortage of the late 1980s. This article describes an RN extender program that used nursing students to provide care that did not require the expertise of an RN. In evaluating the program, observations were made in four categories: (1) direct care, (2) indirect care, (3) unit duties, and (4) personal. A minimum of 400 to a maximum of 1,200 observations were made at each study interval. Data analysis revealed that with the help of clinical assistants, both RNs and licensed practical nurses (LPNs) showed an increase in direct patient care activities. RNs demonstrated an eight percent increase in the time spent on assessments, teaching and family support, which was one of the goals of the program.

There are two tables presented in the article. The first provides an overview of the clinical assistants and RNs hired over a three-year period. The second identifies total nursing time, both RN and LPN, and includes both direct and indirect patient care activities. There is an eight-item bibliography. The article presents an effective nurse extender program.

DeGroot, H. A. (1994). Patient classification systems and staffing: Part 1, Problems and promise. *Journal of Nursing Administration* **24(9):43–51.**

Current methods of linking patient classification systems (PCS) to staffing have been used unevenly and with mixed results. Conflicts arising from the use of PCS for staffing have been resolved at the bargaining table and in the regulatory arena. This article offers a new way to conceptualize and evaluate current methods of staffing with PCS. Adjusting day-to-day staffing according to patient care requirements is not a new concept, but it is one that is vastly underused as an effective management tool. A direct relationship between patient care requirements and staffing is the quintessence of professional staffing models and is the benchmark sought by professional, regulatory, accrediting, and collective bargaining groups. Distinguishing the two direct methods of PCS staffing according to the levels of concern or focus of patient care requirements adds clarity to the process of PCS-related staffing. One approach relies on time standards for individual patients, whereas the other considers the care requirements for the patient population as a whole. Conceptualizing PCS staffing approaches in the new manner allows for a way of comparing and contrasting these methods. Both approaches assume valid and reliable patient classification tool ratings, but they are fundamentally different in the way that staffing projections are made. Although these differences are seldom appreciated, they have significant implications for budget compliance and the overall acceptability of PCS-related staffing programs.

The most common direct method of PCS-related staffing may be aptly called the individual patient time (IPT) model. This approach involves the use of standard time estimates for each patient care level, expressed in minutes, full-time equivalents, or hours per patient day (HPPD). As such, these time standards represent the productive (direct) hours required to care for a given patient at a particular care level or patient category. The article details a different method of PCS-driven staffing. This approach, which relies on valid and reliable ratings of individual patient care requirements and that further considers patient care needs collectively, as an entire group, is said to address many of the inherent shortcomings of the IPT method. As a promising alternative to the IPT approaches, the population care requirements model, avoids some of the more problematic estimation errors in staffing while preserving adequate staffing flexibility.

Two tables are presented: One depicts an individual patient time model; the second, a matrix of medical surgical patient classification system staffing. There is an eleven-item bibliography.

DeGroot, H. A. (1994). Patient classification systems and staffing: Part 2, Practice and process. *Journal of Nursing Administration* **24(10):17–23.**

Part 2 describes further a promising new method of patient classification system (PCS)-related staffing. The population care requirements (PCR) model acknowledges the dynamic interactive nature of the patient care requirement. Using this method, staffing needs increase or decrease according to critical increments rather than in a fixed linear fashion. In addition, although the PCR model also relies on valid and reliable PCS ratings of individual patient care requirements, it is less subject to the more noticeable effects of inaccurate ratings. Because staffing requirements are expressed for the patient group as a whole, the influence of measurement error is minimized. In addition, the PCR model depends on an explicit budgetary relationship as an essential component of staffing projections. When this approach is used, both a minimum and a maximum budget benchmark are clearly identified to ensure that care standards and financial targets are met.

Three tables are presented: One provides a sample calculation of an average PCS level; the second, a matrix of medical–surgical patient classification system staffing; and the third explicates keys to successful implementation of the model. There is a three-item bibliography. The PCR shows promise as a flexible and utilitarian method of staffing that is congruent with professional goals.

Detwiler, C., and Clark, M. J. (1995). Acuity classification in the urgent care setting. *Journal of Nursing Administration* **25(2):53–61.**

In 1991, a California medical center began development of a classification system to be used in six urgent care centers. Patient classification is a method for categorizing patients into acuity levels that reflect the amount of direct and indirect nursing care required. The urgent care classification system was seen as a means of defining the patient population, increasing the accuracy of nursing workload assessments, and allocating staff based on patient care requirements. Appropriate allocation of staff is defined as matching staff time and expertise to patient need.

Three tables are presented in the article. The first presents acuity classification categories. The second includes sample indicators for acuity factors 1–4. Table three displays the mean range of nursing time spent per acuity level. The figures present variation in average patient volume and acuities by day and shift and the number of registered nurse and licensed vocational nurse staff assigned based on day-to-day and shift-to-shift variation in patient volume and acuity. There is a four-item bibliography. Two appendixes are presented: Sample calculations of basic staffing needs and sample calculation of staff mix. The use of the acuity system described in this article has led to recognition of the many aspects of urgent care that nurses are qualified to carry out independently or under the direction of medically approved protocols.

Etheridge, P. (1985). The case for billing by patient acuity. *Nursing Management* **16(8):38–41.**

This article suggests that the most effective way to accumulate data related to the actual cost of nursing care based on the patient's acuity is to accumulate it according to case mix using a patient acuity billing system. Nursing service is the most important marketing source of any health care institution. Consumers, as well as physicians, expect quality from the nursing department. Consumers want a concerned, caring staff and physicians want knowledgeable professional nurses who can collaborate in a meaningful manner.

Four tables are presented that depict conventional budget and staffing for one week, patient distribution by acuity, percentage of allocation of total nursing department expenses, and an acuity charges spreadsheet. There is a six-item bibliography. The article provides support for the perspective that accurate information is like money in the bank—especially when that information is used to provide rationale for budgetary decisions related to staffing.

Flood, S. D., and Diers, D. (1988). Nurse staffing, patient outcome and cost. *Nursing Management* **19(5):34–43.**

This article reports the results of a study that explored the question: "What effect do nurse staffing levels have on patient complications, acuity levels, length of stay, and cost, when controlling for diagnosis-related groups (DRGs)?" This study identified two DRGs in which nurse staffing levels made a difference in the length of stay. Current research has focused only on costs of nursing per DRG, the implication being that the higher the cost, the more nursing care was consumed. The question still remains as to whether the nursing resources consumed lower the length of stay for these particular DRGs. Nurse staffing levels make a difference in patient outcome in areas that can be translated directly into benefits to the hospital. This is especially true of units that have an elderly, chronically ill patient population. By reducing complications, acuity levels, and length of stay through adequate care, nurses potentially can save hospitals a great deal of money. It behooves hospital administrators to develop more attractive compensation packages and increase nursing service budgets for the hiring and retention of more qualified nurses. When units cannot maintain an adequate level of nursing staff, patients suffer from lack of care and hospitals suffer financially from increased lengths of stay.

Five tables are included in the article: a description of full-time equivalent staffing levels by unit, complications by unit, length of stay for specified DRGs, and net revenue and loss for a three-month period. A fifteen-item bibliography is included. This article presents empirical support for the value of nursing to the economic welfare of patients as well as health care institutions.

Fralic, M. A. (1998). How is demand for registered nurses in hospital settings changing? In *Strategies for the Future of Nursing,* **edited by E. O'Neil and J. Coffman. San Francisco: Jossey-Bass.**

The chapter notes that additional research on nurse staffing models is required to determine which models are most effective. Fralic notes the overall supply of nursing professionals is able to meet the needs of hospitals in the short term, regarding the overall number of RNs. Fralic indicates the need to educate more nurses at the baccalaureate level to meet the greater complexity of patients. As nursing practice changes, nurses will be under increased stress to differentiate the practice of associate- and baccalaureate-prepared RNs. This additional requirement will mean significant changes in the hospital team and the deployment of nurses to outpatient units. Acute care nurses, and the hospital itself, will be revolutionized as nursing's efficacy in the delivery of health care services is determined when compared with other providers. Professional nursing will be required to have a full understanding of and to lead the aforementioned health care transition.

The chapter includes a twenty-one-item bibliography. There are two figures: full-time equivalent RNs in community hospitals (1985–1995) and U.S. nursing personnel percentage change by category, September 1994–1995. In addition, two tables are included: recommendations on staffing and quality in hospitals and a contemporary approach to staffing configuration.

Francese, T., and Mohler, M. (1994). Long-term care nurse staffing requirements: Has OBRA really helped? *Geriatric Nursing* **15(3):139–141.**

This article calls for reform in the nursing home industry through public support for adequate reimbursement and by requiring that funds be used to provide adequate care. Gerontological nurses working together to demonstrate the importance of adequate staffing can become the driving force for change.

One graphic presents an overview of current law and proposed nurse staffing standards. The article includes a three-item bibliography. The authors call for nursing to unite in the professional association to work to advance the importance of adequate staffing.

Freitas, C., Helmer, F. T., and Cousins, N. (1987, September/October). The development and management uses of a patient classification system for a high-risk perinatal center. *Journal of Obstetrical Gynecological and Neonatal Nursing* **16(5):330–38.**

This article enforces the value and importance of using a patient classification system for staffing units with frequently changing census and varying patient acuity. The article describes the processes used to develop a system, the importance of identifying direct and indirect patient nursing care activities, and the importance of using the classification system in a timely manner to meeting changing staffing needs.

This article contains five figures outlining patient care activities, direct and indirect care time sheet, staffing and nursing care evaluation questionnaire, and sample computerized staffing recommendations. The article also has two tables identifying risk factors. No bibliography is included. The article supports projecting staffing needs on a shift-by-shift basis and having a patient classification system that can be adapted to the changing needs of the nursing unit.

Gardner. K. (1991). A summary of findings of a five-year comparison of primary and team nursing. *Nursing Research* **40(2):113–117.**

The purpose of this study was to add to the previous evaluations of primary nursing by comparing primary and team nursing on quality of nursing care, nurse retention and distress, and costs during a four-year period. This study supports the founders of primary nursing who advocated primary nursing as a delivery system to promote professional practice and to facilitate the nurse patient relationship. Primary nursing produces higher quality nursing care than team nursing. The effect of primary nursing on staff also was favorable. Once the primary nurses became comfortable with the new delivery system, their stress level scores dropped and were no greater than team nurses. The cost reduction realized was attributed to three factors: fewer nurse administrators on primary units, higher patient-to-staff ratio, and less use of agency nurses.

The article has four tables. The first presents means and standard deviations of total quality of patient care scale scores for primary and team nursing by phases. The second displays hospital stress rating scale and nursing support scale mean scores by phases for primary and team. The third table shows the percentage of retention of RN staff after one, two, and three years primary versus team nursing. The fourth presents cost per patient per day by phases. The article includes a forty-two-item bibliography. The article points out the critical value of institutional support to the success of primary nursing.

Grohar, M. E., Myers, J., and McSweeney, M. (1986). A comparison of patient acuity and nursing resource use. *Journal of Nursing Administration* 16(6):19–23.

The authors of this study sought to develop a model for estimating direct nursing care requirements related to the patient's functional needs. The objectives were to provide a structure to calculate direct nursing hours; provide the basis for calculating the cost of nursing hours; provide a structure to determine the level of caregiver or mix of caregivers needed for a given level of patient acuity; identify areas of possible study to increase efficiency of nursing care delivery; and begin to identify the variety of variables inherent in a predictive model to arrive at a specific staff mix for each diagnosis-related group (DRG). The study identified the inherent variable in a structure to determine direct nursing care in relation to a population of patients representing different functional requirements. Nursing resource use, as described in this study, is widely fluctuating, based on acuity levels, length of stay, and the inherent requirements of particular DRG categories. Functional requirements of the hospitalized patient explain nursing resource use.

The article has six tables and one figure that detail categories and possible categories of nurse patient direct care experiences. The tables depict DRGs and mean length of stay, average hours of direct care, cost of direct nursing care, and cost over length of stay. Also presented are mean resource use in minutes by acuity level; acuity level and category and specific mean resource use by DRG categories. The article has a six-item bibliography. The article notes that although the cost of nursing services can be calculated, the ideal skill mix remains undetermined.

Halloran, E. J. (1983). RN staffing: More care—less cost. *Nursing Management* 14(9):18–22.

The study reported in this article, which was conducted at a large metropolitan acute care Veterans Affairs (VA) hospital is part of an overall research plan intended to incorporate a concept of nursing having face validity in a model for nurse staffing. This pilot study intended to determine whether staff nurses on two typical nursing units can use the nursing diagnosis framework to assess the nursing needs of their patients and to describe the relationship between nursing diagnoses and the time a nurse spends with a patient. The results were surprising to the author. One ward with predominantly (72 percent) RNs operated with fewer staff and more patients than a similar ward with a staff comprised of 40 percent RNs, 40 percent aides, and 20 percent LPNs. The cost of the predominantly registered nurse staff was less than on the alternate ward. When care on the wards was measured using the nursing diagnosis and nursing process concepts, the small but largely RN staff gave the more effective care.

The article includes eight charts: (1) an exhibition of nursing diagnoses; (2) a system model of the nursing process; (3) a matrix of the most frequently occurring nursing diagnoses found in 103 VA patients during 806 patient days; (4) a detailing of the ten highest correlation coefficients between VA patients' nursing diagnoses and the direct care time provided to them; (5) a categorization of nursing diagnoses by Maslow's Hierarchy of Need Theory; (6) two explications of mean correlation coefficients between direct care time and five Maslow's Hierarchy of Need strata; and (7 and 8) the average daily staff and financial data for VA hospital study units. The article has a four-item bibliography. This article provides support for the perspective that "quality" and qualification of nursing staff may be of more value in meeting patient needs as well as decreasing the cost of providing nursing care.

Harvey, G. (1998). Two sides of a coin. *Nursing Standard* 21(13):19–21.

In this article, *Nursing Standard* focuses on the significance of the adequately prepared nurse to high-quality patient care. The article reports on a "snapshot" survey of fifty-five medical wards undertaken by the Royal College of Nursing. The survey indicated that wards are so understaffed that nurses believe they are unable to deliver quality patient care. The article notes patient care is suffering as evidenced by anecdotal comments from nurses who took part in the survey.

The article has no bibliography. The article contains five figures: charts indicating planned number of staff per shift and the average number of beds per staff scheduled for each shift. The article also includes tables of responses to the questions: "Are patients ever put at risk due to short staffing?"; "How does your ward deal with staff absence?"; and "How often is patient care compromised by short staffing?"

Heinemann, D., Lengacher, C. A., VanCott, M. L., Mabe, P., and Swymer, S. (1996, October). Partners in patient care: Measuring the effects on patient satisfaction and other quality indicators. *Nursing Economic$* 14(5):276–285.

This article compares specific quality of care outcomes patient satisfaction, patient medication errors, falls, and intravenous (IV) infections in both control (total patient care) and pilot (Partners in Patient Care [PIPC]) nursing units. The study took place during 18 months, and analysis of data demonstrated a higher level of satisfaction with care on the pilot unit regarding patient satisfaction items: courtesy of all nursing staff, perceptions of staff treatment of family and visitors, and perception of needs being met in a timely manner. No significant differences between units were noted in the number of falls, medication errors, and IV infections. However, when the ratio of these events to patient days was examined, a significant difference was noted between the pilot and control units in the medication error ratio and fall ratio. This article contains four charts, three outlining analysis of variance (ANOVA) comparisons of patient satisfaction and one chi-square analysis of percentage of agreement on patient satisfaction. The article has a fifty-item bibliography. The article tends to diminish the significance of comparable outcomes between pilot and control units in favor of the measurable difference in three areas of patient satisfaction.

Helt, E. H., and Jelinek, R. C. (1988). In the wake of cost cutting, nursing productivity and quality improve. *Nursing Management* 19(6):36–48.

This article reports on a study that analyzes more than eight million patient days in the Medicus National Data Base (MNDB) and that represents one of the most extensive examinations of the effect of recent cost-cutting on productivity and quality. Even in the significant drop in length of stay, and the attendant increase in patient acuity, productivity and quality both improved. Fewer nursing hours were used to care for these patients. Remarkably, quality also improved.

The article contains one table—Medicus NPAQ hospital characteristics. Five charts show the ratio of hours per workload index, percentage change in quality scores, RNs as percentage of direct care staff, mean patient acuity, and average length of stay in Medicus NPAQ hospitals. The bibliography contains two items. The article holds out hope of great promise and opportunity.

Hess, R. G. (1998). Measuring nursing governance. *Nursing Research* 47(1):35–42.

Although studies have measured variables such as job satisfaction, autonomy, professionalism, turnover, leadership styles, and cost-effectiveness, no consistent correlations have been identified between shared governance models and outcomes. This article seeks to define and develop an instrument to measure the governance of hospital-based nurses. The 88-item Index of Professional Nursing Governance (IPNG) was developed to measure professional nursing governance of hospital-based nurses. Psychometric properties were tested with 1,162 registered nurses from ten hospitals.

Content validity after item generation was .95, using Popham's average congruency procedure. Six factors explained 42 percent of the variance with intercorrelations between .43 and .67. All subscales had a high degree of internal consistency (alpha .87 to .91); test–retest reliability was .77.

Construct validity testing showed that scores between shared governance and traditionally governed hospitals varied significantly. A correlation was identified between scores on the IPNG and the Hague and Aiken Index of Centralization. The results of this study support the validity of the 88-item IPNG as a reliable instrument for measuring the distribution of professional nursing governance of hospitals.

The article contains twenty-three citations. The article also has three tables: Characteristics and hospital IPNG scores; intercorrelations between factor subscales; and similar items from factor-derived subscale, personnel.

Hinshaw, A. S., Verran, J., and Chance, H. (1977, April). A description of nursing care requirements in six hospitals. *Community Nursing Research,* 261–83.

Health care is undergoing a number of changes from a variety of perspectives. Trends toward the provision of specialized care by the health profession along with an associated consumer movement directed toward that care have been identified. In addition, fewer resources are being devoted to the delivery of health care in some settings and nursing managers are being asked to provide rationale for their assignment of staff.

This study is descriptive in nature and sought to determine the need for higher registered nurse-to-licensed professional or vocational nurse and nursing assistant ratio in university hospitals. This issue is seen as part of a larger issue of nursing and health care personnel supply and demand.

The article contains a seventeen-item bibliography and one figure, which depicts Perrow's three-stage technological model and its adaptation for nursing technology. There are eleven tables in the article: (1) major characteristics of the six hospitals surveyed; (2) distribution of patient days by hospital and clinical service; (3) summary of actual optimal and relative efficiency estimates by category of patient classification scale; (4) mean value of nursing care required in emotional category across six hospitals by clinical service; (5) mean values for nursing care requirements in the treatment and medical order category across six hospitals by clinical service; (6) mean values for nursing care requirements in the vital signs category across six hospitals by clinical service; (7) mean values for nursing care requirements in feeding category across six hospitals by clinical service; (8) mean value of nursing care requirements in hygiene category across six hospitals by clinical service; (9) mean values of nursing care requirements in activity category across six hospitals by clinical service; (10) total mean value of nursing care required per patient day across six hospitals by clinical service; and (11) nursing care requirements of five hospitals in comparison to university hospital requirements.

Huston, C. L. (1996). Unlicensed assistive personnel: A solution to dwindling health care resources or the precursor to the apocalypse of registered nursing? *Nursing Outlook* 44(2):67–73.

Through an extensive review of the literature this article points out the driving force behind work redesign in the health care system is economical in nature. The authors include some of the recommendations made by the experts for controlling use of unlicensed assistive personnel (UAP):

- Well-designed studies that measure patient outcomes, cost-effectiveness, and work satisfaction are needed to understand the effects of UAP use in nursing care delivery systems.
- Research is also needed to more clearly determine work intensity and acuity relationships so that need and use can be identified and attached to nursing services.
- Titles and job descriptions of UAP must be established.
- Standards for ongoing supervision and periodic verification of UAP competency must be established.

- Implementation of any new practice model must be preceded by an understanding of the present environment, a clear notion of the desired outcomes, and a definition of how to move the organization from the present environment to the desired outcome.
- Job descriptions must be developed by health care agencies that clearly define the roles and responsibilities of all categories of caregivers.
- The organization structure must facilitate RN evaluation of UAP job performance and encourage UAP accountability to the RN.
- There must be adequate program development in leadership and delegation skills for RNs before UAP are introduced.
- Uniform training and orientation programs for UAP must be established to ensure that preparation is adequate to provide at least minimum standards of safe patient care.
- Organizational education programs must be developed for all personnel to learn the roles and responsibilities of different categories of caregivers.

The article has no graphics, but includes a forty-eight-item bibliography. The article calls for the nursing profession to use empirical data to validate its cost-effectiveness in maintaining quality client care.

Joint Commission on the Accreditation of Healthcare Organizations. (1998). *Addressing Staffing Needs for Patient Care: Solutions for Hospital Leaders.* **Oakbrook Terrace, IL: Joint Commission on the Accreditation of Healthcare Organizations.**

This book includes discussion of a variety of topics found within the Joint Commission on the Accreditation of Healthcare Organizations (JCAHO) standards on personnel: defining the number, qualifications, and competencies of staff needed to carry out an organization's mission; providing and ensuring the continued provision of competent staff members; creating a work environment that promotes self-development and learning; ensuring the orientation, education, and competency of all staff. The book does not include information on standards related to personnel with clinical privileges.

The book is divided into four sections: staffing: its challenges and Joint Commission standards; questions and answers about staffing; the survey of staffing requirements; and case studies: design of staffing systems. An appendix containing staffing-related standards from the *Comprehensive Accreditation Manual for Hospitals* is also included. The book has a fifty-seven-item bibliography.

Jung, F. D., Pearcey, L. G., and Phillips, J. L. (1994). Evaluation of a program to improve nursing assistant use. *Journal of Nursing Administration* **24(3):42–47.**

A workload redistribution program was implemented at a 547-bed acute care regional referral center. The purpose of the program was to establish better use of nursing assistants; catalysts for the program included a lack of RN employment applicants and heavy workload demands on existing RNs. The program enabled RNs to delegate more patient care activities to nursing assistants. Variables for study were selected on the basis of reported outcomes of transformational nursing leadership. Therefore, the workload redistribution program was developed within the framework of transformational nursing leadership. Transformational leadership occurs when the RNs and nursing assistants interact to raise one another to higher levels of motivation and development. It was proposed that educating the RNs about an aspect of leadership—specifically, the art and science of delegation—would benefit them in their role and benefit nursing assistants as the two groups interact. Based on the study findings, the program successfully increased the amount of work RNs delegate to nursing assistants, while maintaining patient satisfaction, nurse job satisfaction, and the quality of nursing care. The data show that some improvements in quality and satisfaction may have occurred as a result of the program. Such improvements are reasonable to expect, given that more time and effort are being devoted to the delivery of basic physical and nutritional care, a major factor affecting patient satisfaction. Findings from the evaluation of the program indicate that RN workload can be decreased and quality of care and patient satisfaction improved by increasing nursing assistant use. Furthermore, nursing assistant productivity can be increased by educating RNs about aspects of leadership. Increased nursing assistant use has no seemingly adverse effects on RN job satisfaction.

The article has one figure, which presents the scores of RNs pre- and postimplementation of the redistribution program, and a fourteen-item bibliography. This article presents a program for changing the focus of RNs from working primarily as sole practitioners to functioning as managers of patient care.

Kostovich, C. T., Mahneke, S. M., Meyer, P. A., and Healy, C. (1994). The clinical technician as a member of the patient-focused healthcare delivery team. *Journal of Nursing Administration* **24(12):32–38.**

This article reports on work to evaluate the ancillary and nursing services of an Illinois hospital to determine whether selected components could be coordinated to optimize resource use and maximize patient satisfaction. After much discussion, the decision was made to develop the role of the clinical technician. The goal of the clinical technician program was to eventually achieve budget neutrality (i.e., revenue equals expense) that was not predicted to occur until two years after the program's inception.

Four figures are included in the article: criteria for task selection; a clinical technician interview sheet and general skills list; and a clinical technician criterion checklist: venipuncture for obtaining blood specimen. The article has a fourteen-item bibliography. The overall goal of the work presented in this article is to decrease full-time equivalents in the ancillary services while increasing the total number in the division of nursing, with a net increase of zero or less as efficiencies are realized.

Kovner, C., and Gergen, P. J. (1998). Nurse staffing levels and adverse events following surgery in U.S. hospitals. *IMAGE: Journal of Nursing Scholarship* **30(4):315–321.**

Attempts in the United States to control health care expenses have often resulted in a decrease in the number of nurses providing care. However, there have been few, if any, empirically based attempts to evaluate those activities. This article explores the relationship between nurse staffing and a variety of untoward occurrences that are thought to be nursing-sensitive. The methodology controls for hospital characteristics in 589 acute care hospitals in ten states.

A strong inverse relationship between RNs providing care and postsurgical urinary tract infections was identified. The researchers also found an inverse relationship between staffing and post-op pneumonia. In addition, a statistically significant inverse relationship was identified between the number of RNs and thrombosis after major surgery. These results provide direction for nurse managers in the redesign and restructuring of the nursing workforce.

This article has thirty-nine references. The article contains five tables: states and number of hospitals in sample; frequency and percentage of hospital characteristics; mean, standard deviation, and range of hospital staffing measures; relationship of nurse staffing to adverse events; and mean and standard deviations of adverse events per 100 surgical patients.

Lamkin, L. R., and Sleven, M. (1991). Staffing standards: Why not? A report from the ONS Administration Committee. *Oncology Nursing Forum* **18(7):1241–43.**

The Oncology Nursing Society notes that there are no means by which to ensure that the initial staffing standards are met or to determine whether these standards, when followed, are appropriate. Staffing standards do not lend themselves to clear-cut expectations for nurse-to-patient ratios. Outcome data cannot be quantified because the clarity necessary for development of measurable criteria is lacking. To incorporate hard-and-fast rules for staffing disallows the multitude of factors that inevitably face each manager as he or she endeavors to provide the optimum in both practice and performance. Some of the factors that determine staffing levels are the skill and knowledge levels of the nursing staff, the accessibility of ancillary service personnel, the practice behaviors of physicians, and the intensity level of the service needed. Each manager's ability to assess a unit with respect to these factors and others will enable appropriate decision making.

The article contains two figures and two tables. They provide information related to selected factors for consideration in determining staffing levels and a sample of hypothetical clinical staffing on a thirty-bed unit. The average number of budgeted full-time equivalent positions on a thirty-bed medical surgical oncology unit are presented along with considerations for using survey data. A nine-item bibliography is included. This article, although dated, presents an excellent perspective on issues to be considered in developing a staffing matrix.

Leape, L. (1994) Error in medicine. *Journal of the American Medical Association* **272(23):1851–57.**

This article describes the incidence of iatrogenic injury to patients. The author explains the human factors contributing to errors and postulates that a high percentage of errors are potentially preventable if changes are made in how root cause is identified; how the identification of problems and the faulty systems (rather than individuals) potentiating those problems is encouraged; and how work processes are changed to prevent problems in the future.

This article contains a thirty-six-item bibliography. There are no tables, graphs, or figures.

McClure, M. L., Poulin, M. A., Sovie, M. D., and Wandelt, M. A. (1983). *Magnet Hospitals: Attraction and Retention of Professional Nurses.* **Kansas City, MO: American Nurses Association.**

This monograph focuses on the reasons that nurses stay in their jobs and are satisfied with them by seeking to answer two main study questions:

- What are the important variables in the hospital organization and its nursing service that create a magnetism that attracts and retains professional nurses on its staff?
- What particular combination of variables produces models of hospital nursing practice in which nurses receive professional and personal satisfaction to the degree that recruitment and retention of qualified staff are achieved.

To answer the aforementioned questions, the survey obtained the perceptions of directors of nursing and staff nurses.

One appendix to the monograph is included that provides a description of study materials and procedures.

McDonald, I., and Muller, A. (1998, March). *The Staffing Crisis in Nursing Homes: Why It's Getting Worse & What Can Be Done About It.* **Washington, DC: Service Employees International Union.**

A staffing crisis exists in nursing homes and it is increasing. Short staffing reduces the quality of care received by residents, develops a hazardous environment for caregivers, and leads to certified nurse aide turnover rates in excess of 100 percent. A number of trends aggravate this situation. Acuity levels have risen in nursing homes, but staffing levels have not increased accordingly.

Additionally, nursing homes feel increasing stress because of prospective payment systems and managed care. As a result, staffing levels are inadequate.

Improving the quality of care in nursing homes will demand that there are enough staff to sufficiently meet resident's needs; staff that are fairly compensated, experienced, and well trained; and a safe working environment. The article recommends the following:

- Specific minimum staffing ratios for all caregiving staff,
- Staffing standards linked to acuity,
- Disclosure of staffing ratios,
- Higher wages and better benefits for nursing home workers,
- More training and better supervision for certified nurse aides, and
- Moving forward with the ergonomics standard proposed by the Occupational Safety and Health Administration.

This document reiterates the commitment of the Service Employees International Union to working with policymakers to implement these recommendations so that those who care for seniors and persons with disabilities who require long-term care can provide them with the high-quality services they deserve.

This publication has a twenty-two-item bibliography but no tables, graphs, or figures.

McHugh, M. L., and Dwyer, V. L. (1992). Measurement issues in patient acuity classification for prediction of hours in nursing care. *Nursing Administration Quarterly* 16(4):20–31.

Patient acuity has long been used as a factor in nursing efforts to staff patient care units with the number of nursing hours required to provide appropriate, high-quality nursing care to individual patients. This article presents a short history of patient acuity and its definition. The study reported here focuses on how the method utilized in acuity measurement affects utility of the concept for research and hospital nurse staffing. The authors note that in addition to patient care needs and nurse staffing patterns, a hospital's organizational and task structures affect the consumption of nursing time.

In addition to four figures, a sidebar is included that details Torgersen's ten categories of nursing activity. The figures portray a distribution of hours of nursing care that is "normal" over the four levels of care along with an ideal distribution produced by a "perfect" patient classification system. An additional figure superimposes the normal distribution on the ideal distribution. Finally, a typical distribution of hours of care by actual classification with the actual distribution of hours of nursing care superimposed is presented. The article has a fourteen-item bibliography. This article supports the use of patient acuity classification systems to explain the consumption of nursing time.

McHugh, M., West, P., Assatly, C., Duprat, L., Howard, L., Niloff, J., Waldo, K., Wandel, J., and Clifford, J. (1996, April). Establishing an interdisciplinary patient care team. *Journal of Nursing Administration* 26(4):21–27.

This article describes how an interdisciplinary team of physicians and RNs used enhanced communication and collaboration efforts to improve the quality of care—in the face of increasing acuity and decreasing length of stay—on a thirty-bed gynecological surgery unit. The hospital was also participating in a restructuring initiative, Strengthening Hospital Nursing; A Program to Improve Patient Care, funded by the Robert Wood Johnson Foundation and Pew Charitable Trusts. Without changing staff mix, scheduling patterns, or commitment to primary nursing, this collaborative approach has resulted in improved quality of care and shortened length of stay for patients. At the same time, the interdisciplinary team approach and formalized patient care rounds have also more actively engaged clinical nurses in planning processes, provided opportunities to discuss contingency plans for patient care, optimized knowledge and efficiency of care through clinical teaching, and optimized the benefits of expertise of more experienced clinicians. Findings also include more comprehensive pre- and postoperative follow-up of patients, smoother delivery of care, consistent standards of care, and opportunities for professional growth for nursing staff. The article makes a strong case for increased use of the nurse as primary patient caregiver in working to meet quality and cost containment issues within health care facilities.

This article contains one figure outlining the goals of integrated practice and one table outlining changes in length of stay over a two-year period. The article has a twenty-six-item bibliography.

McKibbin, R. C. (1990). *The Nursing Shortage and the 1990: Realties and Remedies.* **Kansas City, MO: American Nurses Association.**

This book provides a thorough analysis of all aspects of the existing nursing shortage. This shortage affects all those who require health care, virtually the entire U.S. population. The author calls for immediate action to remedy the situation.

The book contains numerous charts, tables, and figures. The survey tool also is included.

McLaughlin, F. E., Thomas, S. A, and Barter, M. (1995). Changes related to care delivery patterns. *Journal of Nursing Administration* **25(5):35–46.**

This study investigated the restructuring of nursing care services in acute care hospitals. The study focused on the restructuring of nursing care delivery models, RN skill-mix trends, assignment of nonnursing personnel to the nursing department, use of unlicensed assistive personnel (UAP), and RN role changes in health care delivery systems using UAP. In acute care hospitals, this restructuring process has led to changes in care delivery models, in the RN skill mix, in the use of nonnursing personnel and in the use of UAP. These changes indicate the need for nursing administration to establish well-planned in-service orientation programs for professional staff nurses. To prepare staff for the changes in their practice responsibilities, nursing administrators must assume a proactive stance. Nursing administrators must assist RNs in dealing with the change process, encourage their participation in planning role changes, and evaluate the outcomes associated with the changes in redesigned nursing care systems.

The article has one table on the use of care delivery models in specialty areas. The article also has eleven figures, including number of licensed beds; corporate health systems; service area population; RN skill mix; topics included in in-service; orientation of UAP; cost of in-service; and RN role changes related to leadership, communication, teaching, and evaluation. This article points out the implications for nursing practice and education of health care system restructuring. The article has a twenty-seven-item bibliography.

Meissner, J. E., and Carey, K. W. (1994, July). How's your job security? *Nursing,* **94:33–38.**

This article reports the results of a poll on hospital restructuring and downsizing. Ninety-five percent of respondents reported that the nursing staff mix has changed in their hospitals in the past two years. The typical respondent to this survey is a medical surgical staff nurse with fifteen years' nursing experience and nine years' seniority at his or her current hospital. Most respondents (forty-four percent) work in cities, whereas twenty-eight percent work in suburban areas, twenty-one percent in small towns, and seven percent in rural areas. The four regions of the United States were represented proportionally. Only one percent came from Canada.

Four sidebars are included that provide an overview of the results of the poll and the demographics of respondents. The only graphic presents results in various regions of the United States. The article has no bibliography. The authors note that the poll was a self-selecting survey and that generally the more worried someone is the more likely he or she is to speak up.

Mintzberg, H. (1996, July August) Musings on Management. *Harvard Business Review*, 61–67.

This article outlines ten proposals or principles that contradict many of the current management and organizational practices in place. The author looks at organizations as circles with management in the center and those who do the work as those on the perimeter. The author proposes that top and central management have difficulty seeing the realities that exist outside the organization, whereas those doing the bulk of the work have a relatively clear view of what happens inside and outside the organization. In environments where middle mangers have been eliminated (those who are capable of seeing what needs to happen in the center to facilitate the productivity on the outer edges), much of the decision making reduces or obstructs productivity and creativity.

The author identifies nursing as a model for management because, rather than intervening and dramatically altering work processes or staffing configurations when things go wrong, nurses (and women) continuously assess, nurture, and monitor work by moving about the organization. Nursing management is likened to the "craft" style of management that works to inspire rather than empower and that is based on mutual respect rooted in common experience and deep understanding.

The article contains no bibliography, figures, charts, or tables.

Mitchell, P. H., Heinrich, J., Moritz, P., and Hinshaw, A. S., eds. (1997). Outcome measures and care delivery systems conference. *Medical Care: Official Journal of the Medical Care Section, American Public Health Association*, 35 (11 Supplement).

This supplement reports on an American Academy of Nursing conference on outcomes measures and care delivery systems. The purposes of the conference were as follows:

- Identify and clarify outcome indicators currently shown to be sensitive to organizational factors in care delivery,
- Identify promising indicators for further measurement development or incorporation into studies of care delivery systems, and
- Develop research and policy recommendations regarding measurement development and incorporation of measures into existing data sources.

The supplement contains the following:

Mitchell, P. H., Heinrich, J., and Moritz, P. and Hinshaw, A.S.	Outcome measures and care delivery systems: Introduction and purposes of conference.
Aiken, L. H., Sochalski, J., and Lake, E. T.	Studying outcomes of organizational change in health services.

Outcome Indicators and Variations in Organization of Care Delivery

Mitchell, P. H., and Shortell, S. M.	Adverse outcomes and variations in organization of care delivery.
Henry, S. B., and Holzemer, W. L.	Achievement of appropriate self-care: Does care delivery system make a difference?
Murdaugh, C.	Health-related quality of life as an outcome in organizational research.

Patrick, D. L.

Finding health-related quality of life outcomes sensitive to health-care organization and delivery.

Rosenthal, G. E., and Shannon, S. E.

The use of patient perceptions in the evaluation of health-care delivery systems.

Hester, N. O., Miller, K. L., Foster, R. L., and Vojir, C. P.

Symptom management outcomes: Do they reflect vacations in care delivery systems?

Theoretical and Methodological Issues in Linking Organizations and Outcomes

Perrin, E. J., and Mitchell, P. H.

Data, information and knowledge: Theoretical and methodological issues in linking outcomes and organizational variables: Introduction.

Brooten, D.

Methodological issues linking costs and outcomes.

Hogan, A. J.

Methodological issues in linking costs and health outcomes in research on differing care delivery systems.

Lamb, G. S.

Outcomes across the care continuum.

Shaughnessy, P. W., Crisler, K. S., Schlenker, R. E., and Arnold, A. G.

Outcomes across the care continuum: Home health care.

Moving Measurement into Practice

Mitchell, P. H., Heinrich, J., Moritz, P., and Hinshaw, A. S.

Measurement into practice: Summary and recommendations.

Murphy, E. C. (1993). *Cost-Driven Downsizing in Hospitals: Implications for Mortality.* **Amherst, NY: E. C. Murphy.**

This study assesses the effects of cost-driven downsizing on Health Care Financing Administration Medicare reported mortality data for hospitals. The study involves 281 general acute care hospitals and 502 health care executives within those hospitals. Hospitals that made across-the-board staffing cuts of 7.5 percent or more during fiscal year 1990, or that were at an average staffing level of 3.35 full-time equivalent staff per adjusted occupied bed or below for that fiscal year, were more likely to experience an increase in mortality and morbidity during 1990 than other hospitals in the sample, including those hospitals that had downsized using less global measures. This study suggests that hospital restructuring, although vital for continued success in the increasingly competitive marketplace, should be approached cautiously and should use a patient-focused methodology that eliminates waste and provides adequate staffing for direct care.

Neidlinger, S. H., Bostrom, J., Stricker, A., Hild, J., and Zhang, J. Q. (1993). Incorporating nursing assistive personnel into a nursing professional proactive model. *Journal of Nursing Administration* **23(3):29–37.**

This article reports on a study in one 560-bed, unionized university medical center where the RN vacancy rate averaged sixty-eight per month throughout the hospital in 1989 to 1990. Nurses from local registries and traveling nurses were used to meet the shortfall. Nursing staff and administrators believed that this approach reduced the continuity and quality of patient care and increased demands among the "regular" staff. Significant increases in personnel costs were also documented. When unlicensed assistive personnel are used, it is essential that the distinction between nonprofessional and professional responsibilities is clear. If the institutional decision is to hire additional unprepared and inexperienced nursing assistive personnel, additional didactic and orientation time for the assistive personnel before they begin to administer care in the unit would be advised. A nurse educator or other designated individual could develop a more intensive, formalized program and also could provide interim clinical supervision of forthcoming nursing assistive personnel. The costs of such orientation of novices need to be forecast and weighed against hiring already certified nursing assistants.

The article has seven tables: (1) personnel costs per patient (in dollars), (2) registry costs per patient day in actual dollars, (3) a comparison of patient satisfaction with nursing care on experimental and control units before and after intervention, (4) a comparison of proportions (in percent) of RNs' work activities (observations for experimental and control units), (5) nursing assistive personnel work activities (observed and reported after implementation), (6) RN job satisfaction, and (7) conditions necessary for the effective integration of nursing assistive personnel to support the professional practice model (as reported by staff RNs). The article has a seventeen-item bibliography. This article reiterates the position of the Tri-Council, which notes the clearer the RN's expectations and direction of assistive personnel, the less likely it is that problems regarding role distinction will occur and the greater the potential for appropriate use of nursing assistive personnel to support the professional nurse's practice.

Parrinello, K. M. (1987). Accounting for patient acuity in an ambulatory surgery center. *Nursing Economic$* 5(4):167–172.

This article presents the results of a study (*Amalgam of nursing acuity, DRGs, and costs*, NLN Publication 1986) that replicates the work by Sovie, VanPutte, Tarcinale, and Stunden to measure variable nursing workload in an ambulatory surgery center using Strong Memorial Hospital's inpatient classification instrument. The effective management of nursing resources requires a link between the costs of services and the patients who receive them. Nursing patient classification systems (PCSs) provide a means to measure nursing workload by patient day or by patient visit in an ambulatory setting. Nursing workload indexes can then be developed and used in the direct calculation of nursing care costs by individual patients. This study represents efforts to measure and monitor the cost of nursing care associated with ambulatory surgery patients. The study demonstrated the feasibility of using an inpatient classification system in an ambulatory surgery center as a methods for categorizing patients into groups of similar nursing resource requirements. In addition, the study demonstrated that the methods for a self-report time study proposed by Sovie et al. can be replicated to establish a database for assigning valid nursing care hours per category of acuity as measured by the nursing patient classification system.

The article contains six tables that include patient classification indicators (assessment/observation, functional, nursing intervention, and special needs) for medical surgical, obstetric/gynecological, and pediatric patients. The article also has frequency distributions of study sample by classification category and service. Nursing care time (in minutes) for three classes of patients is presented along with total nursing time requirements for each of the aforementioned classes. Finally, nursing care hour requirements based on time study findings are displayed. The article has a three-item bibliography. The article provides support for the use of PCSs in ambulatory settings, noting the importance of effective and efficient management of nursing resources in every aspect of health care.

Plati, C., Lemonidou, C., Katostaras, T., Mantas, J., and Lanara, V. (1998). Nursing manpower development and strategic planning in Greece. *IMAGE: Journal of Nursing Scholarship* 30(4):329–333.

This national study cataloged employed nursing personnel and nursing students to evaluate the nursing requirements of the Greek population beyond the year 2000 to design a nursing resource master plan to meet those needs in Greece. First, a questionnaire was distributed to enlist all nursing personnel. Second, personnel requirements were estimated according to the population of each of the country's regions. Third, a master plan for ensuring the development of nursing personnel to the year 2010 was developed. The authors found that there is a serious shortage of RNs in the Greek health services resulting in a decrease of nursing care quality.

The article contains three tables detailing current nursing personnel in all health services and students in nursing schools (November 1993), the distribution of population and nursing personnel by geographic region, and a development planning summary for Greece. The article has an eighteen-item bibliography.

Powers, P. H., Dickey, C. A., and Ford, A. (1990). Evaluating an RN/coworker model. *Journal of Nursing Administration* **20(3):11–15.**

In 1988, the University of Kentucky Hospital established a nurse extender model to cope with diminishing RN resources. After a year and a half of operation, the model was evaluated in terms of training costs, retention, personnel costs, RN and coworker satisfaction, and effect on quality of care. Perhaps the most important criterion evaluated was the effect of the coworker model on the quality of patient care and on staffing based on patient acuity, census, and skill mix. RNs can now increase their patient load from one RN per four patients to one RN per six or seven patients by using a coworker model. The article presents a number of conclusions and recommendations:

- Applicants for coworker positions can be recruited and cost-effectively trained. Applicants need not be employed until able to successfully complete the training program. Tuition and book payment incentives are good, but expecting students to support themselves during the training period seems to produce a more committed employee.
- Staff who have been properly prepared will use the model as it was defined. Managers must understand and accept the concept of the RN–coworker partnership and must find ways to properly schedule these pairs. If not, the concept is not properly implemented and coworkers are used in the traditional nursing assistant role.
- Sick time, overtime, and the use of on-call nurses increase when fewer RNs and more nonprofessional staff are employed. Exploration of use of alternative shifts or overlapping shifts may help to reduce overtime and allow nurses time needed for documentation. With a decrease in the minimum number of RNs, an increasing need exists for management support on evening and night shifts.
- The coworker model is a strategy that will allow beds to stay open and will increase the RN productivity level. In hospitals where high census and high acuity demand that beds remain open, this model is cost-effective.
- RNs can adjust to the coworker model. With decreased peer support and increased patient ratios, the deleterious effect on primary nursing is frustrating to the RN.
- The coworker sees himself or herself as a valuable, important part of the health care team.
- Quality of patient care must be closely monitored and analyzed. RNs need to increase their ability to supervise ancillary staff and monitor patient outcomes.

The article contains one figure, a nursing assistant assignment sheet. The article has two tables, a comparison of hours per relative index of workload and a matrix of quality monitoring scores. The article has no bibliography. Although the program was continued, questions arose about the quality of patient care being provided.

Prescott, P., and Philips, C. Y. (1988, January). Gauging nursing intensity to bring costs to light. *Nursing and Health Care* **9(1):17–22.**

This article addresses the importance of isolating and measuring nursing service delivery to account for the cost of nursing services not only based on volume but also on complexity. Introduction of a new measure of intensity of nursing services, the patient intensity for nursing index (PINI), can assist in that process. The PINI is a tool used by the nurse caring for the patient because that nurse is the only individual with all the current information relevant to that patient. The PINI is a non disease-specific tool that a hospital can apply to all patient populations for research on intensity of nursing care provided, for assistance in staffing and quality assurance, and for estimating the cost of nursing care for selected patient groups. An additional benefit for nursing administrators is the ability to document the need for more appropriate staffing.

This article contains five figures depicting conceptual dimensions of the PINI, complexity of care by volume of nursing, hours of care by acuity level for selected patient classifications, reliability for PINI, and the PINI itself. The article has an eighteen-item bibliography. This article reinforces the need and value of including PINI measurements to identify and support nursing's contributions to patient care.

Prescott, P., Phillips, C. Y., Ryan, J., and Thompson, K. O. (1991, Spring). Changing how nurses spend their time. *IMAGE: Journal of Nursing Scholarship* 23(1):23–28.

This article reports on work sampling studies used to examine how nurses spend their time and to relate nurses' time to the shortage of nursing practice in hospitals. Included are proposals for improving delivery of nursing care, as well as possible pitfalls. Inappropriate use of nurses is divided into two areas: (1) doing the work of other departments and lesser trained individuals and (2) underuse of the skills and abilities of the RN through limited decision-making ability or from doing work that should be done by others. Proposals for improving delivery of care include developing assistive nursing personnel, developing new types of workers to provide nonclerical support to RNs, implementing labor-saving technologics, and restructuring the role of RNs. The article concludes that although all four approaches have potential benefits; they must be implemented in such a way as to not replace the RN with lesser skilled individuals and ultimately fragment nursing care. More and better professional care of patients, not simply more nurses, more assistants, and other changes to replace nurses, will go a long way toward solving the chronic problems of nurse shortage.

This article has four tables comparing RN salaries, salaries for other occupations, outcomes of work sampling studies, and changes in the distribution of hospital beds. One chart outlines the options for improving delivery of nursing care in hospitals. The article has a fifty-three-item bibliography. Although the article was written in early 1991, forecasting of methodologies to replace RNs and anticipated pitfalls of using these approaches have proved accurate.

Prescott, P., Ryan, J. W., Soeken, K. L., Castorr, A. H., Thompson, K. O., and Phillips, C. Y. (1991). The patient intensity for nursing index: A validity assessment. *Research in Nursing and Health* 14:213–21.

This article reports on the psychometric assessment of a new measure of nursing intensity, The patient intensity for nursing index (PINI). Four dimensions are included: severity of illness, dependency on the nurse for care, complexity of care, and time. Standard patient classification systems have not necessarily appreciated the value of nursing intensity—the complexity of decision making that accompanies the skill level at which care is provided. This study evaluated the value of including nursing intensity measures and found internal consistency and reliability of these measures and also that staff nurses found it to capture "the essence of nursing intensity." The research also found that the PINI produces an estimate of total nursing care delivered rather than an estimated need for care (staffing system).

This article contains two tables—one outlining reliability between caregiver nurses and one describing correlation coefficients for the six hypotheses used to assess validity of the PINI. The article has a twenty-four-item bibliography. Use of the PINI as part of patient classification systems should more accurately reflect the care needs and staffing needs on patient care units.

Riley, W., and Schaefers, V. (1983). Costing nursing services. *Nursing Management* 14(12):40–43.

This study reviewed data from calendar year 1982 using Curtin's model for identifying costs on the basis of diagnosis-related groups (DRGs). The Curtin model proposed assigning dollar figures to a patient classification system and thereby converting the patients' intensity index to a monetary amount to calculate total nursing costs. The study demonstrated that it is possible to separate nursing costs from the room rate and base these costs on the intensity of nursing care. This finding underscores the necessity for the nursing administrator to separate nursing costs from the room rate, because it is only then that nursing costs can legitimately be compared with other hospital department costs. This study shows that (1) nursing costs can be measured on the basis of patient severity; (2) it is possible to examine the relationship between nursing costs and DRG classification; and (3) the proportion of nursing costs to total hospital charges is relatively small.

Three charts and one graph present resource requirements and the cost of nursing care for four selected DRGs, nursing costs and total charges, and a frequency distribution for length of stay by DRG. The article has a six-item bibliography. This study provides a readily replicable methodology for identifying nursing as a revenue center.

Rosenbaum, H. L., Willert, T. M., Kelly, E. A., Grey, J. F., and McDonald, B. R. (1988). Costing out nursing services based on acuity. *Journal of Nursing Administration* 18(7,8):10–16.

Because nursing is a personnel intensive, high-budget service, nurse managers have recognized the need to monitor costs and identify potential areas for change to decrease expenditures. The article notes that an effective acuity system can be used to not only efficiently determine appropriate staffing but also to estimate direct nursing costs under diagnosis-related group (DRG) reimbursement. This article describes a method for using patient acuity to determine direct nursing costs on a DRG.

Four charts present the average hours worked, the number of patients and their acuity levels, and a comparison of total average acuity per number of patients with actual staff hours per number of patients on a specified ward. The article has a six-item bibliography. This continuing education offering provides details on examining the relationship between acuity and nurse staffing.

Russo, J. M. K., and Lancaster, D. R. (1995). Evaluating unlicensed assistive personnel models: Asking the right questions, collecting the right data. *Journal of Nursing Administration* 25(9):51–57.

This article provides nurse executives and researchers with insight into the five major areas to consider in the evaluation of the unlicensed assistive personnel (UAP) model. These include program cost-effectiveness, customer satisfaction, patient outcomes, and evaluation of the success of both the training and model implementation processes. If an organization is to remain competitive, current rapid changes in health care require nurse executives to make quick but informed decisions. A number of new roles and care delivery models will continue to be invented and investigated to respond to health care changes. The debate regarding the need to establish a differentiated practice model is sure to be rekindled, and the evolving changes in health care will require that nurses continue to work toward more clearly defining the essence of nursing practice.

Five figures are included in the article. The first includes demographics and implementation process evaluation questions. Training program evaluation data, questions, and methods are displayed. Evaluation of program cost-effectiveness is displayed. RN and UAP satisfaction questions as well as those related to research are provided. The article has an eighteen-item bibliography. A need exists for nurse executives to have the ability to gather evaluation data about the effectiveness of new and emerging delivery systems and to share that information with peers. This article provides a means for gathering these critical data.

Ryten, E. (1997). *A Statistical Picture of the Past, Present and Future of Registered Nurses in Canada.* Ottawa, ON: Canadian Nurses Association.

This report was commissioned by the Canadian Nurses Association (CNA) and urges immediate action to avert a shortage. It indicates that Canada could face a shortage of up to 113,000 RNs by

2011 unless nursing, government, and educators act now. The study predicts a shortage because of increased demands from the growing aging population, an aging nursing workforce, and decreasing nursing school enrollment.

The report makes seven recommendations:

1. Every effort should be made to facilitate the entry into nursing practice of newly qualified RNs.
2. The number of places for the study of nursing should be increased to enable at least 10,000 or more graduates per year.
3. CNA should conduct a study to determine this number.
4. The recruitment of students into nursing should have the goal of an increase in intake of younger students who will have a long working life ahead of them.
5. CNA should try to ascertain how the employment prospects of new RNs since 1991 were affected by the budget constraints of the past five years.
6. CNA should monitor the nursing workforce in relation to evolving need or demand from now on.
7. CNA should monitor inputs to and outputs from nursing education programs to see whether the numbers are in line with the projections in this report.

The report has no bibliography. However, sources are listed for a number of the twenty-four tables:

1. Total health expenditures summary table;
2. Real total health expenditures by category of expenditures;
3. Trends in total number of RNs compared with number of RNs employed in nursing, Canada, 1966–1996;
4. Numbers of RNs employed in nursing, full-time and part-time, Canada, 1985–1996;
5. Employed RNs by sex, Canada, 1985–1996;
6. Place of employment of RNs employed in nursing, Canada, 1985–1996;
7. Age of RNs employed in nursing, Canada, 1966–1996: numeric distribution;
8. Age of RNs employed in nursing, Canada, 1966–1996: percentage distribution;
9. Number of RNs in 1980 and 1995 by single year of age (all RNs);
10. Age at graduation in nursing by year of graduation: RNs in 1995 who graduated in 1980 or later;
11. Comparison of age at graduation of RNs who graduated before 1980 and RNs who graduated in 1980 or later, graduates of 1993;
12. Number of students graduating in nursing by type of initial qualification, Canada, 1963–1996, and first-time takers of RN licensing examinations, 1985–1997;
13. Derivation of future demand for nursing services in Canada, 2011;
14. Number of RNs who were registered in 1995 and who will still be registered in 2011 (retention/survival rates 1995 to 2011);
15. Joint impact of retention as an RN and lower rates of employment for older RNs;
16. New registrations, 1985–2010;
17. Projected entrants to nursing, 1995–2010, by year of qualification and age in 2011;
18. Projected number of RNs in 2011 by age;
19. Projected number of RNs employed in nursing in 2011;
20. Summary of projections of future supply of RNs in Canada by age, 2011;
21. Comparison of age of RNs in 1980, 1995, and projected 2011;
22. Employment prospects for nurses, 2011;
23. Number of licensed practical nurses, Canada, 1982–1996; and
24. Immigration and emigration of RNs; Comparison of number of first-time registrants from other countries with number of RNs requesting transfer of credentials.

Sherman, J. J., and Jones, C. B. (1995). The bottom line: Determining costs to allocate nursing resources. *Nursing Policy Forum* 1(4):14–17, 39–40.

The purpose of the study in this article is to determine relationships among cost, acuity, and length of stay at four southeastern hospitals. In addition, the study examines potential cost advantages individual hospitals may have for certain ranges of patient acuity and length of stay; beyond those ranges, hospitals may encounter inefficiencies that could make them less competitive in certain patient markets. Findings show that nursing costs depend on patient acuity and length of stay mix at a particular hospital. For example, direct and total nursing costs change with patient acuity levels. In addition, for a given length of stay, hospitals tend to enjoy a cost advantage only over a narrow range of patient acuity. The study also showed that hospitals with lower billed charges for a given patient acuity level do not keep that advantage across a wide range of length of stays. Clearly, nurses must understand the variables used to determine the cost of care. Knowledgeable providers can offer valuable input into policy decisions that dictate the type and level of services available. With increased layoffs, downsizing, and restructuring issues facing the profession, it is crucial that nurses become proactive in looking for ways to streamline costs while continuing to provide quality, cost-effective care. For optimal success, nurses and other health care providers should recognize and understand the different perspectives held by persons at various organizational levels—from staff nurse to administrator to CEO.

The article has one table, which presents estimated regression equations for the hospitals included in the study, and four figures. Figures present direct nursing costs at acuity levels 1 and 3, billed charges at acuity level 1, and total nursing costs at length of stay 5 as all predicted from the sample data by the Cobb-Douglas function. The article has a seven-item bibliography. The article provides support for the necessity of practitioners understanding the importance of their role in influencing nursing costs.

Shindul-Rothschild, J. (1996). Patient care: How good is it where you work? *American Journal of Nursing* 96(3):22–24.

This article calls for readers to take part in a survey designed to elicit information related to changes in the workplace over the past year and respondents' perceptions of how those changes have affected patient care. The article has no graphics, and the bibliography has seven items. The *AJN Patient Care Survey* is presented following this article with a request for participation by readers.

Shindul-Rothschild, J., Long-Middleton, E., and Berry, D. (1997). 10 keys to quality care. *American Journal of Nursing* 97(11):35–43.

Using responses garnered from the 1996 *AJN* Patient Care Survey, the authors identify trends with which a subset of respondents rate their institutions. The resulting model identifies ten factors that are perceived by the responding RNs as being predictive of the quality of a facility's patient care. The factors are grouped in three areas, structure, process, and outcomes, as follows:

- Structure
  - Reduction in RNs
  - Loss of RN executive without replacement
- Process
  - Time to provide basic nursing care
  - Ability to uphold professional standards
- Outcomes
  - Patient and family complaints
  - Pressure ulcers/skin breakdown

- ◆ Injuries to patients
- ◆ Medication errors

The article contains six figures, which detail how RNs rated patient care in the 1996 survey; factors predicting quality of care; a depiction of structural, process, and outcome factors versus quality of care; and, a quality of care rating versus likelihood to stay in nursing. The article has a twenty-two-item bibliography.

Shogren, E., Calkins, A., and Wilburn, S. (1996). Restructuring may be hazardous to your health. *American Journal of Nursing* 96(11):64–66.

The Bureau of Labor Statistics indicates the rate of injuries and illness among hospital and nursing home workers rose significantly between 1980 and 1992, passing that of workers in private industry, which decreased. The rate among RNs is greater than that for construction workers. It has been determined, however, that some of that increase is attributable to, at least in part, to efforts to control costs such as hospital restructuring activities.

The Minnesota Nurses Association study, conducted in 1995, found a 65.2 percent increase in the number of injuries and illnesses in RNs between 1990 and 1994. During that same time, RN positions were decreased by 9.2 percent within study hospitals. The study substantiates RNs' belief that reductions in staff numbers overall and other skill-mix changes as a result of restructuring negatively affect patient care and also place workers at risk.

The article has two references and no graphs or figures.

Sibbald, B. (1998). The future supply of registered nurses in Canada. *Canadian Nurse* 94(1):22–23.

The article reports on a new study commissioned by the Canadian Nurses Association that urges immediate action to avert a shortage. It indicates Canada could face a shortage of up to 113,000 RNs by 2011 unless nursing, government, and educators act now. The study predicts a shortage caused by increased demands from the growing aging population, an aging nursing workforce, and decreasing nursing school enrollment.

Canada's independent, peer-reviewed study was conducted during the summer of 1997 by Eva Ryten. Ryten used data collected during the past thirty years by a variety of agencies, in a demographic cohort analysis.

Statistics Canada predicts that by 2011, Canada's population will grow twenty-three percent, and the largest percentage of the population will be forty-five years or older. Aging populations are inclined to have the highest health care utilization rate. Hospital utilization rates signify the demand for registered nursing services will grow by forty-six percent by 2011.

The article has no bibliography. However, it includes a chart—RNs: Needed and available projected year 2011—taken from the Statistical Picture of the Past, Present and Future of RNs in Canada, a 1997 Canadian Nurses Association document.

Singh, D. A., and Schwab, R. C. (1998). Retention of administrators in nursing homes: What can management do? *The Gerontologist* 38(3):362–69.

This article notes that nursing home administrator turnover may be forty percent or higher annually. A survey was undertaken and results (a fifty-three percent response rate) were analyzed using factor analysis and multiple regression models. Survey results indicate higher retention is seen when administrators are permitted to act independently, are involved in decision making, are treated fairly, and are provided with reasonable goals. Systems must hire administrators whose values match those of the organization. Administrators in multifacility chains and for-profit organizations appear to have an increased need to include organizational principles that lead to greater job satisfaction within their position descriptions. Skill compatibility appears to be more crucial when the administrator does not have a bachelor's degree.

The article contains a twenty-two-item bibliography. There are six tables: jobs held and years of employment in each position; administrator changes and turnover; multiple regression models; correlation matrix; composition of realized expectations, organizational demands/skill compatibility, and commitment; and significant differences between nursing homes in Michigan and Indiana.

Sochalski, J., Aiken, L. H., Rafferty, A. M., Shamian, J., Muller-Mundt, G., Hunt, J., Giovannetti, P., and Clarke, H. (1998). Building multinational research. *Reflections*, 20–23, 45.

This article reports on the collaborative efforts of nine nurse researchers in five countries. The group has developed an interdisciplinary methodology to identify the relationship of nurse staffing to patient outcomes. The measurement tool, which has been adapted to allow for country-specific aspects, is designed to gather data related to inpatient and long-term mortality rates; hospital readmission rates, and "failure to rescue" rates.

The article includes a fourteen-item bibliography and no graphs or charts.

Spetz, J. (1998). Hospital employment of nursing personnel. *Journal of Nursing Administration* 28(3):20–27.

This article provides information about the use of nursing personnel in California's short-term hospitals from 1977 through 1996. Data from California's Office of Statewide Health Planning and Development (OSHPD) indicate that the average number of hours worked by nursing personnel in short-term general hospitals rose from 1977 to 1996 despite a recent decrease in the number of hospital discharges. Total nursing personnel hours per patient day increased through 1996, and the hours worked by RNs per patient day increased through 1995. Nursing service hours per discharge decreased slightly between 1994 and 1996, probably because of a reduction in the average length of patients' hospital stays. These findings differ from the perceptions of the public and any hospital workers, but several potential explanations exist for the disparity between the perception and the reality of nursing personnel staffing.

Concerns about possible declines in nurse staffing have risen despite the growth of hours worked by nursing personnel. These concerns may be fueled by several factors. First, nursing personnel employment in hospitals grew more slowly between 1994 and 1996 than before 1993. Although growth in the number of hours worked by nursing personnel slowed, the average length of hospital days dropped from 5.8 to 4.5 days. The lower average length of stay is likely to have increased the intensity of care provided to patients during their hospital stays. The lack of a significant increase in hospital use of nursing personnel while care intensity rose may be a cause of the perception that employment is declining. In addition, some hospitals have engaged in highly publicized restructuring of their nursing services, possibly contributing to insecurity among hospital employees. The recent decline in RN, LVN, and aide wages is likely to add to the perception that the use of nursing personnel is decreasing. Finally, an 18.6 percent increase occurred in the number of graduates from basic RN training programs between 1988–1989 and 1993–1994. These new graduates are entering a market with slower growth of RN positions, and they may find it more difficult than they expected to obtain employment in hospitals.

The article contains five figures depicting average hours worked by nursing service personnel and average patient days; per hospital in California from 1977 to 1996. The article also presents average nursing service personnel hours per case-mix adjusted patient day and discharge in California hospitals and the average nursing service personnel hours per case-mix–adjusted patient day in California hospital acute care units in the period from 1984 to 1996. The article has a twenty-five-item bibliography. This article provides a means for understanding the relationship between nursing personnel employment and patient care in California, which will be useful in evaluating possible future changes in staffing in the state and which may be generalizable to other geographic regions.

Strickland, B., and Neely, S. (1995). Using a standard staffing index to allocate nursing staff. *Journal of Nursing Administration* 25(3):13–21.

This article describes the establishment of the Standard Staffing Index as a method to more efficiently determine unit staffing needs and to allocate staff effectively and as a method of correcting inefficiencies and dissatisfaction stemming from use of a patient classification system alone. This tool, used in conjunction with the average patient acuity and the unit census, is a standardized number of nursing hours per patient day based on unit experience. Findings of this new method for determining staffing needs have resulted in more flexibility in allocating nursing resources and budget management.

This article contains four figures depicting sample nursing hours per patient day for a patient care unit, comparison of nursing hours per patient day to census during a seventeen-month period, sample staffing patterns grid, and a sample staffing worksheet. Two tables include analysis of historical data for one patient care unit and a sample productivity report on selected units. The article has a six-item bibliography. This article reports satisfaction with implementation of a Standard Staffing Index tool to more efficiently and effectively determine staffing.

Tillman, H. J., Salyer, J., Corley, M. C., and Mark, B. A. (1997). Environmental turbulence: staff nurse perspectives. *Journal of Nursing Administration* 27(11):15–22.

This article reports the results of a qualitative study that elicited staff nurses' perceptions of the effect of turbulence (i.e., reflecting instability and random change) on their ability to provide quality patient care. The findings indicate the major negative affect that turbulence is having on both nursing practice and patient care.

The article contains a twenty-nine-item bibliography. The article has one table that details participant characteristics.

Tonges, M. C. (1989). Redesigning hospital nursing practice: The Professionally Advanced Care Team (ProACT™) Model, Part 1. *Journal of Nursing Administration* 19(7):31–38.

This article traces the origins of the alternative practice model movement, providing an overview of existing models with a focus on ProACT. The ProACT model contains three roles for nurses: clinical care manager; primary nurse, and licensed practical nurse. One of the essential requirements for successful implementation of this model is a willingness and desire on the part of other departments to break through traditional role barriers and reach out to assist and support the nursing staff in the delivery of patient care. Despite an increased number of full-time equivalent personnel required to implement ProACT, the cost is budget neutral. This is attributable to the change in the mix of employees within the revised staffing patterns. Because licensed practical nurses, aides, and support service hosts are more available than RNs, implementation of an alternative practice model was more realistic than continuing to try to work with a highly RN-intensive staffing plan.

The article has one figure depicting the ProACT model organizational chart and a twenty-six-item bibliography. The model described in this article has been designed to address the need to find ways for fewer RNs to provide high-quality and efficient patient care.

Verran, J. A. (1986). Patient classification in ambulatory care. *Nursing Economic$* 4(5):247–51.

When Giovannetti's (1978) monograph from the division of nursing was published, scant information was included about patient classification in community health settings, such as ambulatory care. Since 1978, minimal classification efforts for outpatient areas have been performed, although not to the extent of efforts in inpatient settings that initiated standards for classification instruments.

Patient classification information appropriately gathered and analyzed offers a productive data bank for a host of nursing decisions affecting patient care economics. A classification instrument that is empirically sound can affect the efficient and cost-effective use of health care resources.

The article contains a nine-piece bibliography and one figure that depicts the three basic components of classification instruments: indicators of care, instrument format, and quantification scheme.

Verran, J., Murdaugh, C., Gerber, R., and Milton, D. (1988). Shortage solutions: Refining the science of managing nursing resources. *Aspen's Advisor for Nurse Executives* 4(3):4–5.

This article reports on the findings of the National League for Nursing's recent newly licensed nurse survey, which shows essentially no unemployment among new RNs. More disconcerting is the finding that nearly one-fourth of the almost 40,000 new RNs surveyed (ninety-eight percent of whom work in hospitals) say they are looking for other nursing positions. Many of the RNs surveyed listed "poor working conditions" among the reasons for being unhappy with their present positions.

The nursing shortage has resulted in both legislators and the public supporting nursing. Professional nursing must capitalize on that publicity and move to enact practice changes that will point out the efficacy and efficiency of RN use.

The article has no bibliography or charts or figures.

Wan, T. T. H., and Shukla, R. K. (1987). Contextual and organizational correlates of the quality of hospital nursing care. *Quality Review Bulletin* 13(2):61–65.

This study was undertaken to determine how selected contextual and organizational variables influence incident rates on medical–surgical units in forty-five community acute care hospitals across the United States. The health care environment of the 1980s is one of increasing concern for cost containment. In such an environment, caution must be exercised to ensure that the quality of health care does not suffer. This study found that the occurrence of patient incidents is influenced by few factors from the hospital's context and organization. Patient acuity is not a significant factor in explaining variations in incident rates (except patient injury), and neither is the number of RNs on staff. The lack of relationship between patient incidents and nursing resource consumption may be explained by variations in the competence of RNs.

The article has one figure, a schematic diagram of the effect of contextual and organizational factors on the quality of nursing care. Four tables are included that provide operational definitions of independent and dependent variables; identify contextual and organizational attributes of the hospitals included in the study; develop a correlation matrix of five types of reported incidents in sixty hospitals; and a multiple regression analysis of incidents by selected predictors. The article has a ten-item bibliography. This article calls for an in-depth examination of the capabilities of individual nurses and their relationship to patient incidents.

Wunderlich, G. S., Sloan, F. A., and Davis, C. K. (1996). *Nursing Staff in Hospitals and Nursing Homes: Is it Adequate?* **Washington, DC: National Academy Press.**

The Institute of Medicine undertook this study as a result of congressional direction to the Secretary of the Department of Health and Human Services in response to concerns expressed related to changes in the health care environment. The committee of experts undertook an objective study during which an extensive body of research and related literature was reviewed and analyzed. A number of hearings were held and written testimony was accepted. Numerous site visits were made, and the committee engaged in discussion with representatives of professional associations, trade organizations, and consumer advocacy groups. In addition, a number of papers (which are included) were commissioned specifically for the committee's review.

As a result of its activities, the committee formulated recommendations in three distinct areas: the level and staffing patterns of nursing personnel to promote quality of care in hospitals; the level and skill mix of nursing personnel in nursing homes to promote quality of care in these facilities; and strategies to reduce work-related injuries and stress.

This publication has an extensive bibliography. Twenty tables and sixteen figures are included.